GALLBLADDER DIET COOKBOOK AND MEAL PLAN

The Ultimate Diet Guide for Gallbladder health. Discover Healing and Tasty low-fat Recipes to enhance your Digestive system.

Olivia Endwell

Disclaimer:

The information provided in this book is for educational and informational purposes only. It is not intended as a substitute for professional medical advice, diagnosis, or treatment. Always seek the advice of your physician or other qualified health provider with any questions you may have regarding a medical condition. Never disregard professional medical advice or delay in seeking it because of something you have read in this book.

The author and publisher disclaim any liability arising directly or indirectly from the use of this book. The information provided is based on the author's best knowledge at the time of writing and is subject to change. The author and publisher do not guarantee the accuracy, completeness, or timeliness of the information presented in this book.

Individual results may vary, and the success of any dietary or lifestyle change depends on various factors, including but not limited to individual commitment and adherence. Before making significant changes to your diet or lifestyle, consult with a qualified healthcare professional.

The views and opinions expressed in this book are those of the author and do not necessarily reflect the official policy or position of any other agency, organization, employer, or company.

TABLE OF CONTENTS

INTRODUCTION

Welcome to the culinary journey designed to transform the way you think about food and the vital organ often overlooked – your gallbladder. In this "Gallbladder Diet Cookbook and Meal Plan," we embark on an exploration that goes beyond recipes; it's a celebration of understanding, health, and delicious possibilities.

Let's kick things off by demystifying the unsung hero of your digestive system – the gallbladder. Nestled beneath your liver, this small pouch plays a crucial role in processing and storing bile, a digestive fluid that aids in breaking down fats. It's like your body's own sous-chef, ensuring that the richness and goodness from your meals are properly absorbed. We'll delve into the intricacies of its function, demystifying the gallbladder's role in your overall well-being.

Why should you care about your gallbladder's well-being? Well, the health of this unassuming organ directly impacts your digestion and nutrient absorption. A poorly managed diet can lead to gallstones, inflammation, and other unpleasant issues. But fear not, as we're here to guide you through the process of crafting a gallbladder-friendly diet that not only supports your digestive system but also tantalizes your taste buds. It's about embracing a lifestyle that nourishes your body and fosters a harmonious relationship with your gallbladder.

Now, you might wonder, "How can a cookbook make a difference?" Our mission is to transform dietary adjustments into a delightful culinary adventure. This cookbook is not just a collection of recipes; it's your companion on a journey towards optimal gallbladder health. Whether you're a kitchen novice or a seasoned chef, we've curated a variety of recipes that are not only easy to follow but also packed with flavors that defy the notion of bland and restrictive diets.

Imagine savoring a delicious blueberry smoothie that not only brightens your morning but also nurtures your gallbladder with every sip. Picture relishing a hearty vegetable stir-fry that fuels your body with essential nutrients without compromising on taste. This cookbook is your passport to a world where nourishing your gallbladder doesn't mean sacrificing the joy of eating.

As you flip through these pages, you'll find a diverse array of breakfasts, lunches, dinners, snacks, and desserts that cater to your taste preferences while aligning with gallbladder-friendly principles. We provide you with the tools to plan your meals strategically, ensuring a balanced and enjoyable gastronomic experience while safeguarding your gallbladder's well-being.

GALLBLADDER DIET BASICS

The health of your gallbladder is intricately tied to the foods you consume. As we delve into the Gallbladder Diet Basics, we aim to demystify the complexities surrounding this vital organ and empower you to make informed dietary choices that foster optimal gallbladder health. Let's embark on a journey of understanding, exploring the nuances of the gallbladder diet, the foods that play a pivotal role, and practical tips for crafting a meal plan that nurtures your digestive system.

Overview of the Gallbladder Diet: Nurturing the Culinary Ecosystem Within

The Gallbladder Diet isn't a restrictive regimen; it's a holistic approach to eating that supports your digestive system. At its core, this diet emphasizes the consumption of nutrient-dense, whole foods while minimizing factors that could burden the gallbladder. We're not talking about a one-size-fits-all approach; instead, it's about tailoring your diet to suit your individual needs and promoting a harmonious relationship with your gallbladder.

Essentially, a gallbladder-friendly diet involves incorporating ample fruits, vegetables, lean proteins, and whole grains. These foods provide essential nutrients while maintaining a balance that supports efficient digestion. Additionally, healthy fats, such as those found in avocados and olive oil, play a crucial role in this diet, as they stimulate the gallbladder to release bile, aiding in the breakdown of fats.

On the flip side, processed foods, excessive saturated fats, and refined sugars are the antagonists in this dietary narrative. These items can contribute to the formation of gallstones and strain the gallbladder. Understanding the principles of the Gallbladder Diet sets the stage for a mindful and nourishing culinary journey, fostering a digestive ecosystem that thrives on wholesome, real foods.

Foods to Include and Avoid: The Culinary Compass for Gallbladder Health

Navigating the world of gallbladder-friendly foods involves distinguishing between the heroes and villains in your plate. Let's start with the champions – fiber-rich fruits and vegetables. These gems not only provide essential vitamins and minerals but also promote healthy digestion by preventing constipation, a factor that can contribute to gallstone formation.

Lean proteins, such as poultry, fish, and tofu, take center stage in the gallbladder-friendly ensemble. These protein sources offer sustenance without burdening your gallbladder with excessive fats. Whole grains, like brown rice and quinoa, bring their fiber and nutrient-rich goodness to the table, aiding in digestion and promoting a sense of fullness.

Now, let's address the culinary foes. High-fat dairy products and fatty meats can be formidable adversaries to your gallbladder. While healthy fats are essential, it's crucial to strike a balance and avoid excessive consumption of saturated and trans fats. Processed foods, laden with additives and preservatives, also find themselves on the blacklist, as they can contribute to inflammation and digestive distress.

Understanding the nuances of these dietary choices empowers you to make informed decisions when crafting your meals. The Gallbladder Diet isn't about deprivation; it's about embracing a variety of nourishing foods that support your digestive system and foster overall well-being.

Tips for Meal Planning with a Focus on Gallbladder Health: A Blueprint for Balanced Nourishment

Meal planning is the linchpin of success in adopting a Gallbladder Diet. It's not just about what you eat; it's about how you structure your meals to promote optimal digestion and gallbladder function. Here, we unravel practical tips to guide you through the art of meal planning with a keen focus on gallbladder health.

Begin by incorporating a rainbow of vegetables into your meals. Not only do they add vibrant colors to your plate, but they also bring a plethora of nutrients and fiber that support digestive health. Aim to fill half your plate with vegetables to ensure a nutrient-dense and gallbladder-friendly foundation for your meals.

When it comes to protein, opt for lean sources such as chicken, fish, beans, and tofu. These proteins provide essential amino acids without the excessive fat content that can burden your gallbladder. Grilled or baked preparations are preferable to frying, minimizing added fats while retaining flavor and texture.

Whole grains should feature prominently in your meal planning. Brown rice, quinoa, and whole-grain pasta offer a rich tapestry of nutrients and fiber, promoting satiety and aiding in digestion. These grains also contribute to stabilizing blood sugar levels, an additional benefit for overall health.

Strategically incorporating healthy fats is key to a gallbladder-friendly meal plan. Include sources like avocados, nuts, and olive oil to stimulate the gallbladder's release of bile without overwhelming it. Pay attention to portion sizes, as even healthy fats can contribute to digestive distress if consumed in excess.

Distribute your meals throughout the day, aiming for smaller, more frequent meals rather than large, heavy ones. This approach prevents the gallbladder from being overloaded with a massive influx of food, reducing the risk of gallstone formation and promoting smoother digestion.

Hydration is a crucial but often overlooked aspect of gallbladder health. Ensure an adequate intake of water throughout the day to support the digestive process and prevent the formation of concentrated bile, which can contribute to gallstone development.

Finally, listen to your body. Pay attention to how different foods make you feel and adjust your meal plan accordingly. Everyone's body is unique, and what works for one person may not work for another. By staying attuned to your body's signals, you can refine your meal plan to suit your individual needs and preferences.

PLANNING YOUR MEALS

In the realm of gallbladder health, meal planning takes center stage, transforming dietary aspirations into tangible, nourishing experiences. "Planning Your Meals" is not merely a logistical exercise; it's a deliberate and thoughtful approach to crafting a culinary journey that aligns with the principles of the Gallbladder Diet. In this exploration, we unravel the intricacies of creating balanced and nutrient-rich meals, understanding the importance of portion control and timing, and offering sample meal plans tailored to diverse dietary preferences.

Creating Balanced and Nutrient-Rich Meals: A Palette of Healthful Choices

Balancing your plate is an art, and when it comes to gallbladder health, it's about more than just aesthetics—it's about fostering an environment that supports optimal digestion and nutrient absorption. A balanced and nutrient-rich meal should be a harmonious composition of macronutrients (carbohydrates, proteins, and fats), fiber, vitamins, and minerals.

Begin by incorporating a variety of colorful vegetables, each hue representing a unique set of antioxidants and phytonutrients. These vegetables not only add vibrancy to your plate but also contribute to digestive health and overall well-being. Aim for a diverse array, from leafy greens to cruciferous vegetables, ensuring a rich tapestry of nutrients.

Lean proteins play a pivotal role in creating a well-rounded meal. Opt for sources like poultry, fish, tofu, or legumes to provide essential amino acids without the excess saturated fats that can burden your gallbladder. Grilled or baked preparations maintain the integrity of the protein without introducing unnecessary fats.

Whole grains should form the backbone of your meal, providing complex carbohydrates and fiber. Brown rice, quinoa, and whole-grain pasta offer sustained energy and contribute to a feeling of fullness, supporting portion control and preventing overeating.

Incorporate healthy fats strategically. Avocados, nuts, and olive oil not only add flavor but also stimulate the gallbladder to release bile, aiding in the digestion of fats. However, moderation is key, as even healthy fats contribute to overall caloric intake.

Consider your meal as a symphony, where each component plays a unique role in creating a balanced and nourishing experience. By embracing a variety of nutrient-dense foods, you not only support your gallbladder but also lay the foundation for sustained energy, satiety, and overall vitality.

Portion Control and Timing: The Rhythmic Dance of Digestive Harmony

Portion control is the silent conductor orchestrating the digestive symphony within your body. It's not about deprivation but rather about tuning in to your body's cues and providing it with the right amount of fuel at the right time. Timing, much like rhythm in music, is crucial in ensuring a smooth and efficient digestive process.

Begin by listening to your body's hunger and fullness signals. Portion control starts with an awareness of your body's needs rather than external cues. Eat when you're hungry, and stop when you're satisfied. This simple yet powerful practice prevents overeating, reducing the strain on your gallbladder and promoting digestive comfort.

Consider the composition of your meals throughout the day. Instead of loading up on a large volume of food in one sitting, distribute your intake across multiple smaller meals and snacks. This approach prevents the gallbladder from being overwhelmed with a sudden influx of food, reducing the risk of gallstone formation and promoting smoother digestion.

Mindful eating goes hand in hand with portion control. Slow down, savor each bite, and pay attention to the flavors and textures. This not only enhances your dining experience but also allows your body to register satiety more effectively, preventing overindulgence.

The timing of your meals also influences gallbladder health. Aim for regular meal times, creating a predictable rhythm for your digestive system. Consistency in meal timing supports the gallbladder's natural processes, optimizing the release of bile and promoting efficient digestion.

Consider the composition of your meals throughout the day. Instead of loading up on a large volume of food in one sitting, distribute your intake across multiple smaller meals and snacks. This approach prevents the gallbladder from being overwhelmed with a sudden influx of food, reducing the risk of gallstone formation and promoting smoother digestion.

Mindful eating goes hand in hand with portion control. Slow down, savor each bite, and pay attention to the flavors and textures. This not only enhances your dining experience but also allows your body to register satiety more effectively, preventing overindulgence.

The timing of your meals also influences gallbladder health. Aim for regular meal times, creating a predictable rhythm for your digestive system. Consistency in meal timing supports the gallbladder's natural processes, optimizing the release of bile and promoting efficient digestion.

In essence, portion control and timing are the unseen choreographers of your digestive ballet. By synchronizing your meals with your body's needs and maintaining a steady rhythm, you create an environment that fosters gallbladder health and overall digestive harmony.

Sample Meal Plans for Different Dietary Preferences: Tailoring the Symphony to Your Tastes

Gallbladder health doesn't subscribe to a one-size-fits-all approach. Recognizing the diversity of dietary preferences, we present sample meal plans that cater to various tastes and lifestyles. Whether you follow a vegetarian, Mediterranean, or low-carb diet, these meal plans serve as templates, illustrating how the principles of the Gallbladder Diet can be adapted to suit your individual preferences.

Vegetarian Meal Plan:

Breakfast:

- Spinach and feta omelet

- Whole-grain toast

- Fresh berries

Lunch:

- Quinoa salad with mixed vegetables and chickpeas

- Greek yogurt with honey

Dinner:

- Lentil soup

- Grilled vegetable skewers

- Brown rice

Snacks:

- Mixed nuts

- Sliced cucumber with hummus

Mediterranean Meal Plan:

Breakfast:

- Greek yogurt with honey and walnuts

- Whole-grain pita bread

Lunch:

- Mediterranean salad with tomatoes, cucumbers, olives, and feta

- Grilled chicken or fish

Dinner:

- Baked salmon with lemon and herbs

- Quinoa pilaf with roasted vegetables

Snacks:

- Hummus with carrot and celery sticks

- Fresh fruit

Low-Carb Meal Plan:

Breakfast:

- Scrambled eggs with spinach and feta

- Avocado slices

Lunch:

- Chicken Caesar salad with extra vegetables

- Olive oil dressing

Dinner:

- Zucchini noodles with pesto and cherry tomatoes

- Grilled shrimp or tofu

Snacks:

- Cheese cubes

- Sliced bell peppers with guacamole

These sample meal plans illustrate the adaptability of the Gallbladder Diet to different dietary preferences. Whether you prefer plant-based options, Mediterranean-inspired flavors, or a low-carb approach, the key is to focus on nutrient-dense, whole foods and maintain a balance of macronutrients. Feel free to customize these plans based on your taste preferences, making the Gallbladder Diet a versatile and enjoyable culinary journey tailored to your unique needs.

SPECIAL CONSIDERATIONS

In the realm of gallbladder health, acknowledging special considerations becomes pivotal as individuals navigate the unique landscape of their well-being. The Gallbladder Diet is not a one-size-fits-all solution; it's a flexible framework that accommodates various circumstances, from weight management goals to specific health conditions. In this exploration, we delve into the nuances of special considerations, addressing the Gallbladder Diet's role in weight management, its adaptability for specific health conditions, and the importance of consulting with a healthcare professional for personalized guidance.

Gallbladder Diet for Weight Management: Nourishing the Body, Balancing the Scale

Weight management is a multifaceted journey that extends beyond calorie counting. When adopting the Gallbladder Diet with a focus on weight management, the emphasis is on crafting a sustainable and nourishing approach that promotes overall health while addressing specific dietary considerations.

The foundation lies in choosing nutrient-dense foods that support gallbladder health and contribute to satiety. High-fiber fruits and vegetables, lean proteins, and whole grains play a pivotal role in creating meals that not only nourish the body but also contribute to a sense of fullness, preventing overeating.

Mindful eating becomes a cornerstone in the pursuit of weight management through the Gallbladder Diet. By paying attention to hunger and fullness cues, individuals can develop a healthier relationship with food. Slow, deliberate consumption allows the body to register satisfaction, reducing the likelihood of overindulgence and supporting weight-related goals.

Strategic inclusion of healthy fats is essential in the Gallbladder Diet for weight management. While healthy fats contribute to satiety, it's crucial to be mindful of portion sizes. Avocados, nuts, and olive oil can be incorporated to enhance flavor and promote digestive health without tipping the scales.

Portion control remains a key aspect of weight management within the Gallbladder Diet. By distributing meals throughout the day and focusing on smaller, more frequent servings, individuals can regulate their caloric intake and support a more balanced approach to weight.

Exercise is a complementary component in the Gallbladder Diet for weight management. Physical activity not only contributes to calorie expenditure but also enhances overall well-being. Whether through cardiovascular exercises or strength training, incorporating regular physical activity aligns with the holistic approach of the Gallbladder Diet.

In essence, adopting the Gallbladder Diet for weight management is about embracing a lifestyle that nourishes the body, supports gallbladder health, and addresses the multifaceted aspects of weight. By combining mindful eating, strategic food choices, portion control, and regular exercise, individuals embark on a comprehensive approach to achieving and maintaining a healthy weight.

Gallbladder Diet for Specific Health Conditions: Adapting to Individual Needs

The Gallbladder Diet is not a one-dimensional protocol; its adaptability extends to addressing specific health conditions. Whether managing conditions like diabetes, high cholesterol, or gastrointestinal issues, the principles of the Gallbladder Diet can be tailored to accommodate individual health needs.

For individuals with diabetes, the emphasis is on regulating blood sugar levels through the strategic selection of carbohydrates. Choosing complex carbohydrates, such as whole grains and legumes, promotes stable blood sugar levels and aligns with the Gallbladder Diet's focus on nutrient-dense foods.

In cases of high cholesterol, the Gallbladder Diet offers a foundation for heart-healthy eating. Prioritizing sources of healthy fats, such as omega-3 fatty acids found in fish and flaxseeds, contributes to cholesterol management while supporting gallbladder health. Additionally, incorporating soluble fiber from fruits, vegetables, and oats aids in lowering cholesterol levels.

Individuals with gastrointestinal issues, such as irritable bowel syndrome (IBS) or inflammatory bowel disease (IBD), can find relief through the Gallbladder Diet's emphasis on whole, easily digestible foods. The inclusion of low-FODMAP (fermentable oligosaccharides, disaccharides, monosaccharides, and polyols) options aligns with the dietary requirements for those with sensitive digestive systems.

Adapting the Gallbladder Diet to specific health conditions involves collaboration with healthcare professionals. A registered dietitian or healthcare provider can offer personalized guidance, considering the nuances of individual health needs and ensuring that the Gallbladder Diet aligns with broader health goals.

Consultation with a Healthcare Professional: Personalized Guidance for Optimal Health

While the Gallbladder Diet provides a valuable framework for digestive wellness, the importance of consulting with a healthcare professional cannot be overstated. Individual health circumstances vary, and seeking personalized guidance ensures that the Gallbladder Diet aligns with specific needs and addresses any underlying health concerns.

Healthcare professionals, including registered dietitians and nutritionists, possess the expertise to tailor the Gallbladder Diet to individual requirements. Through a comprehensive assessment of health history, dietary preferences, and specific health conditions, professionals can offer nuanced recommendations that optimize gallbladder health while addressing broader health goals.

In the context of weight management, healthcare professionals can provide guidance on caloric intake, nutrient distribution, and exercise plans tailored to individual needs. This personalized approach goes beyond generalized recommendations, recognizing the unique factors influencing weight and overall health.

For individuals with specific health conditions, consultation with a healthcare professional ensures that the Gallbladder Diet is adapted to accommodate dietary restrictions, address nutritional deficiencies, and complement existing medical interventions. This collaborative approach enhances the effectiveness of the Gallbladder Diet as a supportive element in managing various health conditions.

Moreover, individuals with pre-existing medical conditions, such as diabetes, cardiovascular issues, or gastrointestinal disorders, benefit from the expertise of healthcare professionals who can navigate the intersection of these conditions with gallbladder health. The Gallbladder Diet becomes a cohesive part of a broader health management strategy under the guidance of these professionals.

BREAKFAST RECIPE

1. Avocado and Spinach Omelet

Prep Time: 10 minutes

Cooking Time: 8 minutes

Serving Size: 1

Ingredients:

- 2 large eggs

- 1/4 cup fresh spinach, chopped

- 1/4 avocado, sliced

- Salt and pepper to taste

- 1 tsp olive oil

Instructions:

1. In a bowl, whisk the eggs until well beaten.

2. Heat olive oil in a non-stick skillet over medium heat.

3. Add chopped spinach to the skillet and sauté until wilted.

4. Pour the beaten eggs over the spinach and let them set for a moment.

5. Place avocado slices on one side of the omelet and season with salt and pepper.

6. Gently fold the omelet over the avocado and cook until the eggs are fully set.

7. Serve hot.

Nutritional Information:

Calories: 320 | Protein: 18g | Carbohydrates: 10g | Fat: 24g | Fiber: 6g

2. Quinoa Breakfast Bowl

Prep Time: 15 minutes
Cooking Time: 15 minutes
Serving Size: 1

Ingredients:

- 1/2 cup cooked quinoa

- 1/4 cup Greek yogurt

- 1/2 cup mixed berries (blueberries, strawberries, raspberries)

- 1 tbsp honey

- 1 tbsp chopped nuts (almonds, walnuts)

Instructions:

1. Cook quinoa according to package instructions.

2. In a bowl, layer cooked quinoa, Greek yogurt, and mixed berries.

3. Drizzle honey over the top and sprinkle with chopped nuts.

4. Mix gently and enjoy.

Nutritional Information:

Calories: 380 | Protein: 15g | Carbohydrates: 55g | Fat: 12g | Fiber: 7g

3. Banana Almond Pancakes

Prep Time: 10 minutes

Cooking Time: 10 minutes

Serving Size: 2 pancakes

Ingredients:

- 1 ripe banana, mashed

- 2 eggs

- 1/4 cup almond flour

- 1/2 tsp baking powder

- 1/2 tsp vanilla extract

- Pinch of salt

- Butter or oil for cooking

Instructions:

1. In a bowl, combine mashed banana, eggs, almond flour, baking powder, vanilla extract, and a pinch of salt. Mix until well combined.

2. Heat a skillet over medium heat and add butter or oil.

3. Spoon the batter onto the skillet to form pancakes.

4. Cook until bubbles appear on the surface, then flip and cook the other side.

5. Repeat until all the batter is used.

6. Serve with your favorite toppings.

Nutritional Information:

Calories: 280 | Protein: 11g | Carbohydrates: 20g | Fat: 18g | Fiber: 4g

4. Berry and Chia Seed Parfait

Prep Time: 15 minutes (plus chilling time)

Cooking Time: 0 minutes

Serving Size: 1

Ingredients:

- 1/2 cup Greek yogurt

- 1/4 cup mixed berries

- 1 tbsp chia seeds

- 1 tbsp honey

- Granola for topping

Instructions:

1. In a glass or bowl, layer Greek yogurt, mixed berries, and chia seeds.

2. Drizzle honey over the top.

3. Refrigerate for at least 2 hours or overnight.

4. Before serving, top with granola for added crunch.

Nutritional Information:

Calories: 320 | Protein: 18g | Carbohydrates: 40g | Fat: 10g | Fiber: 8g

5. Spinach and Feta Breakfast Wrap

Prep Time: 10 minutes

Cooking Time: 5 minutes

Serving Size: 1

Ingredients:

- 1 whole-grain tortilla

- 2 large eggs, scrambled

- 1/4 cup fresh spinach

- 2 tbsp feta cheese, crumbled

- Salt and pepper to taste

Instructions:

1. Heat a tortilla in a dry skillet or microwave until warm.

2. In another skillet, scramble the eggs over medium heat.

3. Add fresh spinach to the skillet and sauté until wilted.

4. Place the scrambled eggs and spinach in the center of the tortilla.

5. Sprinkle feta cheese over the top and season with salt and pepper.

6. Fold the sides of the tortilla and roll it up into a wrap.

7. Serve immediately.

Nutritional Information:

Calories: 340 | Protein: 20g | Carbohydrates: 25g | Fat: 18g | Fiber: 5g

6. Overnight Oats with Almond Butter

Prep Time: 5 minutes (plus chilling time)

Cooking Time: 0 minutes

Serving Size: 1

Ingredients:

- 1/2 cup rolled oats

- 1/2 cup almond milk

- 1 tbsp almond butter

- 1 tbsp chia seeds

- 1/2 banana, sliced

- 1 tsp honey

Instructions:

1. In a jar or container, combine rolled oats, almond milk, almond butter, and chia seeds.

2. Stir well, cover, and refrigerate overnight.

3. In the morning, top with banana slices and drizzle honey over the oats.

4. Mix and enjoy.

Nutritional Information:

Calories: 380 | Protein: 10g | Carbohydrates: 50g | Fat: 16g | Fiber: 9g

7. Smoked Salmon and Avocado Toast

Prep Time: 10 minutes

Cooking Time: 5 minutes

Serving Size: 1

Ingredients:

- 1 slice whole-grain bread, toasted

- 2 oz smoked salmon

- 1/4 avocado, sliced

- 1 tbsp cream cheese

- Fresh dill for garnish

Instructions:

1. Toast the whole-grain bread to your liking.

2. Spread cream cheese on the toasted bread.

3. Arrange smoked salmon slices on top.

4. Place avocado slices over the salmon.

5. Garnish with fresh dill and serve.

Nutritional Information:

Calories: 320 | Protein: 20g | Carbohydrates: 20g | Fat: 18g | Fiber: 5g

8. Sweet Potato and Turkey Sausage Hash

Prep Time: 15 minutes

Cooking Time: 20 minutes

Serving Size: 2

Ingredients:

- 1 sweet potato, diced

- 1/2 lb turkey sausage, crumbled

- 1 bell pepper, diced

- 1/2 onion, diced

- 2 tbsp olive oil

- Salt and pepper to taste

- 2 eggs (optional)

Instructions:

1. In a skillet, heat olive oil over medium heat.

2. Add diced sweet potato and cook until slightly browned and softened.

3. Add turkey sausage, bell pepper, and onion. Cook until sausage is browned and vegetables are tender.

4. Season with salt and pepper to taste.

5. If desired, cook eggs sunny-side-up and place them on top of the hash.

6. Serve hot.

Nutritional Information:

Calories: 450 | Protein: 25g | Carbohydrates: 30g | Fat: 25g | Fiber: 6g

9. Blueberry Almond Smoothie Bowl

Prep Time: 5 minutes

Cooking Time: 0 minutes

Serving Size: 1

Ingredients:

- 1 cup frozen blueberries

- 1/2 banana

- 1/2 cup almond milk

- 1 tbsp almond butter

- Toppings: sliced almonds, chia seeds, fresh blueberries

Instructions:

1. In a blender, combine frozen blueberries, banana, almond milk, and almond butter.

2. Blend until smooth and creamy.

3. Pour the smoothie into a bowl.

4. Top with sliced almonds, chia seeds, and fresh blueberries.

5. Serve immediately.

Nutritional Information:

Calories: 300 | Protein: 8g | Carbohydrates: 40g | Fat: 14g | Fiber: 10g

10. Cottage Cheese and Pineapple Bowl

Prep Time: 5 minutes

Cooking Time: 0 minutes

Serving Size: 1

Ingredients:

- 1 cup low-fat cottage cheese

- 1/2 cup fresh pineapple chunks

- 1 tbsp honey

- 1 tbsp shredded coconut

Instructions:

1. In a bowl, combine cottage cheese and fresh pineapple chunks.

2. Drizzle honey over the top.

3. Sprinkle shredded coconut for added flavor.

4. Mix gently and enjoy.

Nutritional Information:

Calories: 280 | Protein: 25g | Carbohydrates: 30g | Fat: 8g | Fiber: 2g

11. Veggie and Goat Cheese Frittata

Prep Time: 15 minutes

Cooking Time: 20 minutes

Serving Size: 2

Ingredients:

- 4 large eggs

- 1/2 cup cherry tomatoes, halved

- 1/4 cup bell peppers, diced

- 1/4 cup red onion, finely chopped

- 2 tbsp goat cheese

- Salt and pepper to taste

- Fresh herbs for garnish

Instructions:

1. Preheat the oven to 350°F (180°C).

2. In a bowl, whisk the eggs until well beaten.

3. Add cherry tomatoes, bell peppers, and red onion to the bowl. Mix well.

4. Pour the egg mixture into a greased oven-safe skillet.

5. Crumble goat cheese over the top and season with salt and pepper.

6. Bake in the preheated oven for 20 minutes or until the frittata is set.

7. Garnish with fresh herbs and serve.

Nutritional Information:

Calories: 320 | Protein: 18g | Carbohydrates: 10g | Fat: 24g | Fiber: 3g

12. Almond Flour Banana Muffins

Prep Time: 15 minutes

Cooking Time: 20 minutes

Serving Size: 2 muffins

Ingredients:

- 1 cup almond flour

- 1/2 tsp baking soda

- Pinch of salt

- 2 ripe bananas, mashed

- 2 large eggs

- 1/4 cup almond milk

- 1 tsp vanilla extract

Instructions:

1. Preheat the oven to 350°F (180°C) and line a muffin tin with paper liners.

2. In a bowl, mix almond flour, baking soda, and a pinch of salt.

3. In a separate bowl, combine mashed bananas, eggs, almond milk, and vanilla extract.

4. Add the wet ingredients to the dry ingredients and stir until well combined.

5. Spoon the batter into the muffin tin, filling each cup about two-thirds full.

6. Bake for 20 minutes or until a toothpick inserted into the center comes out clean.

7. Allow the muffins to cool before serving.

Nutritional Information:

Calories: 240 | Protein: 8g | Carbohydrates: 20g | Fat: 16g | Fiber: 4g

13. Mediterranean Egg Wrap

Prep Time: 10 minutes

Cooking Time: 5 minutes

Serving Size: 1

Ingredients:

- 1 whole-grain tortilla

- 2 large eggs, scrambled

- 1/4 cup cherry tomatoes, halved

- 2 tbsp feta cheese, crumbled

- 1 tbsp Kalamata olives, chopped

- Fresh basil for garnish

Instructions:

1. Heat a tortilla in a dry skillet or microwave until warm.

2. In another skillet, scramble the eggs over medium heat.

3. Place the scrambled eggs in the center of the tortilla.

4. Add cherry tomatoes, feta cheese, and chopped Kalamata olives.

5. Garnish with fresh basil and fold the sides of the tortilla.

6. Serve immediately.

Nutritional Information:

Calories: 340 | Protein: 20g | Carbohydrates: 25g | Fat: 18g | Fiber: 5g

14. Green Smoothie with Kale and Pineapple

Prep Time: 8 minutes

Cooking Time: 0 minutes

Serving Size: 1

Ingredients:

- 1 cup kale, stems removed

- 1/2 cup pineapple chunks

- 1/2 banana

- 1/2 cup almond milk

- 1 tbsp chia seeds

- Ice cubes (optional)

Instructions:

1. In a blender, combine kale, pineapple chunks, banana, almond milk, and chia seeds.

2. Blend until smooth.

3. Add ice cubes if desired and blend again.

4. Pour into a glass and enjoy immediately.

Nutritional Information:

Calories: 250 | Protein: 8g | Carbohydrates: 40g | Fat: 10g | Fiber: 10g

15. Turkey and Veggie Breakfast Burrito

Prep Time: 15 minutes

Cooking Time: 10 minutes

Serving Size: 1

Ingredients:

- 1 whole-grain tortilla

- 2 large eggs, scrambled

- 2 oz lean ground turkey, cooked

- 1/4 cup bell peppers, diced

- 1/4 cup black beans, drained and rinsed

- Salsa for topping

Instructions:

1. Heat a tortilla in a dry skillet or microwave until warm.

2. In another skillet, scramble the eggs over medium heat.

3. Add cooked ground turkey, diced bell peppers, and black beans.

4. Place the scrambled eggs and turkey mixture in the center of the tortilla.

5. Top with salsa.

6. Fold the sides of the tortilla and serve immediately.

Nutritional Information:

Calories: 380 | Protein: 25g | Carbohydrates: 30g | Fat: 18g | Fiber: 8g

16. Apple Cinnamon Chia Pudding

Prep Time: 10 minutes (plus chilling time)

Cooking Time: 0 minutes

Serving Size: 1

Ingredients:

- 1/4 cup chia seeds

- 1 cup almond milk

- 1/2 apple, diced

- 1/2 tsp cinnamon

- 1 tbsp maple syrup (optional)

Instructions:

1. In a jar or container, combine chia seeds, almond milk, diced apple, and cinnamon.

2. Stir well, cover, and refrigerate for at least 2 hours or overnight.

3. Before serving, drizzle with maple syrup if desired.

4. Mix and enjoy.

Nutritional Information:

Calories: 290 | Protein: 8g | Carbohydrates: 35g | Fat: 14g | Fiber: 14g

17. Egg and Veggie Muffin Cups

Prep Time: 15 minutes

Cooking Time: 20 minutes

Serving Size: 2 muffin cups

Ingredients:

- 4 large eggs

- 1/2 cup cherry tomatoes, halved

- 1/4 cup spinach, chopped

- 2 tbsp feta cheese, crumbled

- Salt and pepper to taste

- Cooking spray

Instructions:

1. Preheat the oven to 350°F (180°C) and grease a muffin tin with cooking spray.

2. In a bowl, whisk the eggs until well beaten.

3. Add cherry tomatoes, chopped spinach, and crumbled feta cheese. Mix well.

4. Pour the egg mixture into the muffin tin, filling each cup about two-thirds full.

5. Bake for 20 minutes or until the egg muffins are set.

6. Allow them to cool before serving.

Nutritional Information:

Calories: 280 | Protein: 16g | Carbohydrates: 8g | Fat: 20g | Fiber: 2g

18. Mango Coconut Chia Parfait

Prep Time: 15 minutes (plus chilling time)

Cooking Time: 0 minutes

Serving Size: 1

Ingredients:

- 1/4 cup chia seeds

- 1 cup coconut milk

- 1/2 mango, diced

- 2 tbsp shredded coconut

- 1 tbsp agave syrup (optional)

Instructions:

1. In a jar or container, combine chia seeds and coconut milk.

2. Stir well, cover, and refrigerate for at least 2 hours or overnight.

3. Before serving, layer chia pudding with diced mango and shredded coconut.

4. Drizzle with agave syrup if desired.

5. Mix and enjoy.

Nutritional Information:

Calories: 350 | Protein: 6g | Carbohydrates: 40g | Fat: 18g | Fiber: 12g

19. Mediterranean Chickpea Scramble

Prep Time: 10 minutes

Cooking Time: 10 minutes

Serving Size: 1

Ingredients:

- 1/2 cup canned chickpeas, rinsed and drained

- 2 large eggs, scrambled

- 1/4 cup cherry tomatoes, halved

- 2 tbsp feta cheese, crumbled

- 1 tbsp fresh parsley, chopped

- 1 tbsp olive oil

- Salt and pepper to taste

Instructions:

1. Heat olive oil in a skillet over medium heat.

2. Add chickpeas and cook for 3-4 minutes until slightly crispy.

3. Add scrambled eggs, cherry tomatoes, and crumbled feta cheese.

4. Cook until the eggs are fully set.

5. Season with salt and pepper.

6. Garnish with fresh parsley and serve.

Nutritional Information:

Calories: 380 | Protein: 20g | Carbohydrates: 30g | Fat: 18g | Fiber: 8g

20. Pomegranate and Walnut Yogurt Bowl

Prep Time: 10 minutes

Cooking Time: 0 minutes

Serving Size: 1

Ingredients:

- 1 cup Greek yogurt

- 1/2 cup pomegranate arils

- 2 tbsp chopped walnuts

- 1 tbsp honey

- Fresh mint for garnish

Instructions:

1. In a bowl, layer Greek yogurt, pomegranate arils, and chopped walnuts.

2. Drizzle honey over the top.

3. Garnish with fresh mint and enjoy.

Nutritional Information:

Calories: 320 | Protein: 20g | Carbohydrates: 25g | Fat: 18g | Fiber: 4g

LUNCH RECIPES

1. Grilled Chicken Salad with Lemon-Tahini Dressing

Prep Time: 15 minutes

Cooking Time: 15 minutes

Serving Size: 2

Ingredients:

- 2 boneless, skinless chicken breasts

- 6 cups mixed salad greens

- 1 cup cherry tomatoes, halved

- 1 cucumber, sliced

- 1/4 red onion, thinly sliced

- 1/4 cup feta cheese, crumbled

Lemon-Tahini Dressing:

- 3 tbsp tahini

- 2 tbsp fresh lemon juice

- 1 tbsp olive oil

- 1 garlic clove, minced

- Salt and pepper to taste

Instructions:

1. Season chicken breasts with salt and pepper, then grill until cooked through.

2. In a large bowl, combine salad greens, cherry tomatoes, cucumber, red onion, and grilled chicken (sliced).

3. In a small bowl, whisk together tahini, lemon juice, olive oil, minced garlic, salt, and pepper to create the dressing.

4. Drizzle the dressing over the salad, toss gently, and top with crumbled feta cheese.

Nutritional Information:

Calories: 400 | Protein: 30g | Carbohydrates: 20g | Fat: 22g | Fiber: 6g

2. Quinoa and Vegetable Stuffed Peppers

Prep Time: 20 minutes

Cooking Time: 30 minutes

Serving Size: 2 peppers

Ingredients:

- 1 cup cooked quinoa

- 2 large bell peppers, halved and seeds removed

- 1 cup black beans, drained and rinsed

- 1 cup corn kernels

- 1 cup cherry tomatoes, diced

- 1/2 cup red onion, finely chopped

- 1 tsp cumin

- 1/2 tsp chili powder

- Salt and pepper to taste

- 1/4 cup fresh cilantro, chopped

Instructions:

1. Preheat the oven to 375°F (190°C).

2. In a bowl, combine cooked quinoa, black beans, corn, cherry tomatoes, red onion, cumin, chili powder, salt, and pepper.

3. Fill each bell pepper half with the quinoa mixture.

4. Place the stuffed peppers in a baking dish and bake for 25-30 minutes or until the peppers are tender.

5. Garnish with fresh cilantro before serving.

Nutritional Information:

Calories: 380 | Protein: 15g | Carbohydrates: 70g | Fat: 5g | Fiber: 12g

3. Lemon Herb Baked Salmon with Roasted Vegetables

Prep Time: 15 minutes

Cooking Time: 20 minutes

Serving Size: 2

Ingredients:

- 2 salmon fillets

- 1 lb mixed vegetables (zucchini, bell peppers, cherry tomatoes)

- 2 tbsp olive oil

- 2 tbsp fresh lemon juice

- 1 tsp dried oregano

- 1 tsp dried thyme

- Salt and pepper to taste

Instructions:

1. Preheat the oven to 400°F (200°C).

2. Place salmon fillets on a baking sheet and surround them with mixed vegetables.

3. Drizzle olive oil and fresh lemon juice over the salmon and vegetables.

4. Sprinkle dried oregano, dried thyme, salt, and pepper evenly.

5. Bake for 20 minutes or until the salmon is cooked through
   and the vegetables are tender.

Nutritional Information:

Calories: 420 | Protein: 30g | Carbohydrates: 20g | Fat: 25g | Fiber:
8g

4. Lentil and Vegetable Soup

Prep Time: 15 minutes

Cooking Time: 30 minutes

Serving Size: 4

Ingredients:

- 1 cup dried green or brown lentils, rinsed

- 1 onion, chopped

- 2 carrots, diced

- 2 celery stalks, chopped

- 3 garlic cloves, minced

- 1 can (14 oz) diced tomatoes

- 6 cups vegetable broth

- 1 tsp ground cumin

- 1 tsp paprika

- 1/2 tsp turmeric

- Salt and pepper to taste

- Fresh parsley for garnish

Instructions:

1. In a large pot, sauté onion, carrots, celery, and garlic until softened.

2. Add lentils, diced tomatoes, vegetable broth, cumin, paprika, turmeric, salt, and pepper.

3. Bring to a boil, then reduce heat and simmer for 25-30 minutes or until lentils are tender.

4. Garnish with fresh parsley before serving.

Nutritional Information:

Calories: 320 | Protein: 18g | Carbohydrates: 55g | Fat: 2g | Fiber: 20g

5. Shrimp and Broccoli Stir-Fry with Brown Rice

Prep Time: 20 minutes

Cooking Time: 15 minutes

Serving Size: 2

Ingredients:

- 1 lb shrimp, peeled and deveined

- 2 cups broccoli florets

- 1 bell pepper, sliced

- 1 carrot, julienned

- 2 tbsp soy sauce

- 1 tbsp sesame oil

- 1 tbsp rice vinegar

- 1 tbsp honey

- 2 garlic cloves, minced

- 1 tsp ginger, grated

- 2 cups cooked brown rice

Instructions:

1. In a wok or skillet, stir-fry shrimp until pink and opaque. Set aside.

2. In the same wok, stir-fry broccoli, bell pepper, and carrot until crisp-tender.

3. In a small bowl, whisk together soy sauce, sesame oil, rice vinegar, honey, minced garlic, and grated ginger.

4. Add cooked shrimp back to the wok, pour the sauce over the mixture, and toss until well coated.

5. Serve over cooked brown rice.

Nutritional Information:

Calories: 420 | Protein: 30g | Carbohydrates: 60g | Fat: 8g | Fiber: 8g

6. Turkey and Vegetable Lettuce Wraps

Prep Time: 20 minutes

Cooking Time: 15 minutes

Serving Size: 4

Ingredients:

- 1 lb ground turkey

- 1 tbsp olive oil

- 1 onion, finely chopped

- 2 garlic cloves, minced

- 1 bell pepper, diced

- 1 zucchini, grated

- 1 carrot, grated

- 1 cup water chestnuts, chopped

- 3 tbsp soy sauce

- 1 tbsp hoisin sauce

- 1 tsp sesame oil

- Butter lettuce leaves

Instructions:

1. In a skillet, brown ground turkey in olive oil until cooked through.

2. Add chopped onion, minced garlic, diced bell pepper, grated zucchini, grated carrot, and chopped water chestnuts. Sauté until vegetables are tender.

3. In a small bowl, mix together soy sauce, hoisin sauce, and sesame oil. Pour over the turkey and vegetable mixture, stirring well.

4. Spoon the mixture into butter lettuce leaves to create wraps.

Nutritional Information:

Calories: 350 | Protein: 25g | Carbohydrates: 20g | Fat: 18g | Fiber: 6g

7. Eggplant and Chickpea Tagine

Prep Time: 20 minutes

Cooking Time: 40 minutes

Serving Size: 2

Ingredients:

- 1 eggplant, diced

- 1 can (14 oz) chickpeas, drained and rinsed

- 1 onion, chopped

- 2 garlic cloves, minced

- 1 can (14 oz) diced tomatoes

- 1/2 cup vegetable broth

- 1 tsp ground cumin

- 1 tsp ground coriander

- 1/2 tsp cinnamon

- Salt and pepper to taste

- Fresh cilantro for garnish

Instructions:

1. In a large pot, sauté diced eggplant, chopped onion, and minced garlic until softened.

2. Add chickpeas, diced tomatoes, vegetable broth, ground cumin, ground coriander, cinnamon, salt, and pepper.

3. Bring to a simmer, cover, and cook for 30 minutes or until the eggplant is tender.

4. Garnish with fresh cilantro before serving.

Nutritional Information:

Calories: 340 | Protein: 15g | Carbohydrates: 60g | Fat: 5g | Fiber: 18g

8. Spinach and Feta Stuffed Chicken Breast

Prep Time: 20 minutes

Cooking Time: 25 minutes

Serving Size: 2

Ingredients:

- 2 boneless, skinless chicken breasts

- 2 cups fresh spinach

- 1/2 cup feta cheese, crumbled

- 1 garlic clove, minced

- 1 tsp olive oil

- Salt and pepper to taste

Instructions:

1. Preheat the oven to 375°F (190°C).

2. In a skillet, sauté fresh spinach and minced garlic in olive oil until wilted. Set aside.

3. Cut a pocket into each chicken breast.

4. Stuff each pocket with the sautéed spinach and crumbled feta cheese.

5. Season the chicken breasts with salt and pepper.

6. Bake for 25 minutes or until the chicken is cooked through.

Nutritional Information:

Calories: 320 | Protein: 40g | Carbohydrates: 5g | Fat: 15g | Fiber: 2g

9. Lemon Dill Greek Salad with Grilled Shrimp

Prep Time: 20 minutes

Cooking Time: 10 minutes

Serving Size: 2

Ingredients:

- 1 lb shrimp, peeled and deveined

- 6 cups mixed salad greens

- 1 cucumber, sliced

- 1 cup cherry tomatoes, halved

- 1/4 red onion, thinly sliced

- 1/2 cup Kalamata olives, pitted

- 1/2 cup feta cheese, crumbled

Lemon Dill Dressing:

- 3 tbsp olive oil

- 2 tbsp fresh lemon juice

- 1 tbsp fresh dill, chopped

- 1 garlic clove, minced

- Salt and pepper to taste

Instructions:

1. Season shrimp with salt and pepper, then grill until pink and opaque.

2. In a large bowl, combine salad greens, cucumber, cherry tomatoes, red onion, Kalamata olives, and grilled shrimp.

3. In a small bowl, whisk together olive oil, lemon juice, chopped dill, minced garlic, salt, and pepper to create the dressing.

4. Drizzle the dressing over the salad, toss gently, and top with crumbled feta cheese.

Nutritional Information:

Calories: 380 | Protein: 30g | Carbohydrates: 20g | Fat: 20g | Fiber: 6g

10. Sweet Potato and Turkey Chili

Prep Time: 20 minutes

Cooking Time: 30 minutes

Serving Size: 4

Ingredients:

- 1 lb ground turkey

- 1 onion, chopped

- 2 sweet potatoes, peeled and diced

- 1 can (14 oz) black beans, drained and rinsed

- 1 can (14 oz) diced tomatoes

- 1 cup corn kernels

- 2 cups vegetable broth

- 2 tbsp chili powder

- 1 tsp cumin

- 1/2 tsp smoked paprika

- Salt and pepper to taste

- Fresh cilantro for garnish

Instructions:

1. In a large pot, brown ground turkey with chopped onion until cooked through.

2. Add diced sweet potatoes, black beans, diced tomatoes, corn, vegetable broth, chili powder, cumin, smoked paprika, salt, and pepper.

3. Bring to a boil, then reduce heat and simmer for 25-30 minutes or until sweet potatoes are tender.

4. Garnish with fresh cilantro before serving.

Nutritional Information:

Calories: 350 | Protein: 25g | Carbohydrates: 45g | Fat: 8g | Fiber: 10g

11. Mediterranean Quinoa Salad with Lemon Vinaigrette

Prep Time: 15 minutes

Cooking Time: 15 minutes

Serving Size: 4

Ingredients:

- 1 cup cooked quinoa

- 1 cucumber, diced

- 1 cup cherry tomatoes, halved

- 1/2 cup Kalamata olives, pitted and sliced

- 1/4 red onion, finely chopped

- 1/2 cup feta cheese, crumbled

Lemon Vinaigrette:

- 3 tbsp olive oil

- 2 tbsp fresh lemon juice

- 1 tsp Dijon mustard

- 1 garlic clove, minced

- Salt and pepper to taste

Instructions:

1. In a large bowl, combine cooked quinoa, diced cucumber, cherry tomatoes, Kalamata olives, red onion, and crumbled feta cheese.

2. In a small bowl, whisk together olive oil, lemon juice, Dijon mustard, minced garlic, salt, and pepper to create the vinaigrette.

3. Pour the vinaigrette over the quinoa mixture and toss gently before serving.

Nutritional Information:

Calories: 320 | Protein: 12g | Carbohydrates: 35g | Fat: 15g | Fiber: 6g

12. Baked Cod with Lemon Garlic Butter Sauce

Prep Time: 15 minutes

Cooking Time: 20 minutes

Serving Size: 2

Ingredients:

- 2 cod fillets

- 2 tbsp olive oil

- 3 garlic cloves, minced

- Zest of 1 lemon

- 2 tbsp fresh lemon juice

- 2 tbsp fresh parsley, chopped

- Salt and pepper to taste

Instructions:

1. Preheat the oven to 400°F (200°C).

2. Place cod fillets on a baking sheet.

3. In a small bowl, mix olive oil, minced garlic, lemon zest, lemon juice, chopped parsley, salt, and pepper.

4. Pour the lemon garlic butter mixture over the cod fillets.

5. Bake for 20 minutes or until the fish is opaque and flakes easily.

Nutritional Information:

Calories: 300 | Protein: 25g | Carbohydrates: 2g | Fat: 20g | Fiber: 1g

13. Chickpea and Vegetable Stir-Fry

Prep Time: 15 minutes

Cooking Time: 15 minutes

Serving Size: 2

Ingredients:

- 1 can (14 oz) chickpeas, drained and rinsed

- 1 cup broccoli florets

- 1 bell pepper, sliced

- 1 carrot, julienned

- 1 cup snow peas

- 2 tbsp soy sauce

- 1 tbsp hoisin sauce

- 1 tbsp sesame oil

- 2 garlic cloves, minced

- 1 tsp ginger, grated

- 2 cups cooked quinoa

Instructions:

1. In a wok or skillet, stir-fry chickpeas, broccoli, bell pepper, carrot, and snow peas until vegetables are crisp-tender.

2. In a small bowl, whisk together soy sauce, hoisin sauce, sesame oil, minced garlic, and grated ginger.

3. Add the sauce to the stir-fry and toss until well coated.

4. Serve over cooked quinoa.

Nutritional Information:

Calories: 380 | Protein: 15g | Carbohydrates: 65g | Fat: 8g | Fiber: 12g

14. Turkey and Sweet Potato Skillet

Prep Time: 15 minutes

Cooking Time: 20 minutes

Serving Size: 4

Ingredients:

- 1 lb ground turkey

- 2 sweet potatoes, peeled and diced

- 1 bell pepper, diced

- 1 onion, chopped

- 2 garlic cloves, minced

- 1 tsp ground cumin

- 1 tsp paprika

- 1/2 tsp cinnamon

- Salt and pepper to taste

- Fresh cilantro for garnish

Instructions:

1. In a large skillet, brown ground turkey with diced sweet potatoes, diced bell pepper, chopped onion, and minced garlic until turkey is cooked through and sweet potatoes are tender.

2. Add ground cumin, paprika, cinnamon, salt, and pepper. Stir well.

3. Cook for an additional 5 minutes until flavors meld.

4. Garnish with fresh cilantro before serving.

Nutritional Information:

Calories: 340 | Protein: 25g | Carbohydrates: 30g | Fat: 15g | Fiber: 6g

15. Avocado and Black Bean Wrap

Prep Time: 10 minutes

Cooking Time: 0 minutes

Serving Size: 2

Ingredients:

- 1 can (14 oz) black beans, drained and rinsed

- 1 avocado, sliced

- 1 cup cherry tomatoes, halved

- 1/4 red onion, thinly sliced

- 2 tbsp fresh cilantro, chopped

- Juice of 1 lime

- Salt and pepper to taste

- 2 whole-grain tortillas

Instructions:

1. In a bowl, combine black beans, sliced avocado, cherry tomatoes, sliced red onion, chopped cilantro, lime juice, salt, and pepper.

2. Warm tortillas in a dry skillet or microwave until pliable.

3. Spoon the black bean mixture onto each tortilla.

4. Roll up the tortillas to create wraps.

Nutritional Information:

Calories: 320 | Protein: 10g | Carbohydrates: 50g | Fat: 12g | Fiber: 14g

16. Pesto Zucchini Noodles with Grilled Chicken

Prep Time: 15 minutes

Cooking Time: 10 minutes

Serving Size: 2

Ingredients:

- 2 zucchinis, spiralized

- 2 boneless, skinless chicken breasts

- 2 tbsp pesto sauce

- 1 tbsp olive oil

- Cherry tomatoes for garnish

- Parmesan cheese for garnish

Instructions:

1. Season chicken breasts with salt and pepper, then grill until cooked through.

2. In a skillet, heat olive oil and sauté spiralized zucchini for 2-3 minutes until just tender.

3. Toss zucchini noodles with pesto sauce.

4. Slice grilled chicken and serve over the pesto zucchini noodles.

5. Garnish with cherry tomatoes and Parmesan cheese.

Nutritional Information:

Calories: 380 | Protein: 30g | Carbohydrates: 10g | Fat: 25g | Fiber: 3g

17. Chickpea and Spinach Stuffed Portobello Mushrooms

Prep Time: 20 minutes
Cooking Time: 20 minutes
Serving Size: 2 mushrooms

Ingredients:

- 4 large Portobello mushrooms, stems removed

- 1 can (14 oz) chickpeas, drained and rinsed

- 2 cups fresh spinach, chopped

- 1/2 red onion, finely chopped

- 2 garlic cloves, minced

- 2 tbsp olive oil

- 1 tsp dried oregano

- 1/2 tsp smoked paprika

- Salt and pepper to taste

- Feta cheese for topping

Instructions:

1. Preheat the oven to 375°F (190°C).

2. Place Portobello mushrooms on a baking sheet.

3. In a skillet, sauté chickpeas, chopped spinach, chopped red onion, and minced garlic in olive oil until spinach wilts.

4. Season with dried oregano, smoked paprika, salt, and pepper.

5. Spoon the chickpea and spinach mixture into each Portobello mushroom.

6. Top with crumbled feta cheese.

7. Bake for 20 minutes or until mushrooms are tender.

Nutritional Information:

Calories: 340 | Protein: 18g | Carbohydrates: 40g | Fat: 15g | Fiber: 12g

18. Teriyaki Salmon and Vegetable Skewers

Prep Time: 20 minutes

Cooking Time: 10 minutes

Serving Size: 2

Ingredients:

- 2 salmon fillets, cut into chunks

- 1 bell pepper, cut into chunks

- 1 zucchini, sliced

- 1 red onion, cut into chunks

- 1/2 cup teriyaki sauce

- 1 tbsp sesame seeds

- Green onions for garnish

Instructions:

1. Preheat the grill or grill pan.

2. Thread salmon chunks, bell pepper, zucchini, and red onion onto skewers.

3. Brush the skewers with teriyaki sauce.

4. Grill for 8-10 minutes, turning occasionally, until salmon is cooked through and vegetables are tender.

5. Sprinkle sesame seeds and garnish with chopped green onions.

Nutritional Information:

Calories: 400 | Protein: 28g | Carbohydrates: 30g | Fat: 18g | Fiber: 6g

19. Cabbage and Turkey Stir-Fry with Ginger Soy Sauce

Prep Time: 15 minutes

Cooking Time: 15 minutes

Serving Size: 2

Ingredients:

- 1 lb ground turkey

- 4 cups shredded cabbage

- 1 bell pepper, thinly sliced

- 1 carrot, julienned

- 2 tbsp soy sauce

- 1 tbsp sesame oil

- 1 tbsp rice vinegar

- 1 tbsp fresh ginger, grated

- 2 garlic cloves, minced

- 2 green onions, sliced

- Sesame seeds for garnish

Instructions:

1. In a large wok or skillet, brown ground turkey until cooked through.

2. Add shredded cabbage, sliced bell pepper, julienned carrot, grated ginger, and minced garlic. Stir-fry for 5-7 minutes until vegetables are tender-crisp.

3. In a small bowl, whisk together soy sauce, sesame oil, rice vinegar, and sliced green onions.

4. Pour the sauce over the turkey and vegetable mixture, toss until well coated.

5. Garnish with sesame seeds before serving.

Nutritional Information:

Calories: 350 | Protein: 30g | Carbohydrates: 20g | Fat: 18g | Fiber: 8g

20. Cauliflower Fried Rice with Shrimp

Prep Time: 15 minutes

Cooking Time: 15 minutes

Serving Size: 2

Ingredients:

- 1 lb shrimp, peeled and deveined

- 4 cups cauliflower rice

- 1 cup frozen peas and carrots, thawed

- 2 eggs, beaten

- 3 tbsp soy sauce

- 1 tbsp sesame oil

- 1 tsp ginger, grated

- 2 green onions, sliced

- Sesame seeds for garnish

Instructions:

1. In a large skillet, cook shrimp until pink and opaque. Set aside.

2. In the same skillet, stir-fry cauliflower rice with peas and carrots until heated through.

3. Push the cauliflower rice to the side, pour beaten eggs into the skillet, and scramble until cooked.

4. Mix the cooked shrimp back into the cauliflower rice and egg mixture.

5. In a small bowl, whisk together soy sauce, sesame oil, grated ginger, and sliced green onions. Pour over the cauliflower fried rice and toss until well combined.

6. Garnish with sesame seeds before serving.

Nutritional Information:

Calories: 380 | Protein: 30g | Carbohydrates: 20g | Fat: 18g | Fiber: 8g

DINNER RECIPES

1. Lemon Herb Baked Chicken Thighs with Roasted Vegetables

Prep Time: 15 minutes

Cooking Time: 25 minutes

Serving Size: 2

Ingredients:

- 4 bone-in, skin-on chicken thighs
- 1 lb mixed vegetables (broccoli, carrots, cauliflower)
- 2 tbsp olive oil
- 2 tbsp fresh lemon juice
- 1 tsp dried oregano
- 1 tsp dried thyme
- Salt and pepper to taste

Instructions:

1. Preheat the oven to 400°F (200°C).
2. Place chicken thighs on a baking sheet and surround them with mixed vegetables.

3. Drizzle olive oil and fresh lemon juice over the chicken and vegetables.

4. Sprinkle dried oregano, dried thyme, salt, and pepper evenly.

5. Bake for 25 minutes or until the chicken is cooked through and vegetables are tender.

Nutritional Information:

Calories: 420 | Protein: 30g | Carbohydrates: 20g | Fat: 25g | Fiber: 8g

2. Quinoa and Salmon Patties with Dill Yogurt Sauce

Prep Time: 20 minutes

Cooking Time: 15 minutes

Serving Size: 2

Ingredients:

- 1 cup cooked quinoa

- 2 cans (7.5 oz each) canned salmon, drained and flaked

- 1/4 cup whole wheat breadcrumbs

- 1/4 cup green onions, chopped

- 1 egg

- 2 tbsp fresh dill, chopped

- 1/2 lemon, zest and juice

- Salt and pepper to taste

Dill Yogurt Sauce:

- 1/2 cup Greek yogurt

- 1 tbsp fresh dill, chopped

- 1 tsp lemon juice

- Salt and pepper to taste

Instructions:

1. In a bowl, combine cooked quinoa, canned salmon, breadcrumbs, green onions, egg, chopped dill, lemon zest, lemon juice, salt, and pepper.

2. Form the mixture into patties.

3. In a skillet, cook the patties over medium heat until golden brown on both sides.

4. For the dill yogurt sauce, mix together Greek yogurt, chopped dill, lemon juice, salt, and pepper.

5. Serve the salmon patties with the dill yogurt sauce.

Nutritional Information:

Calories: 380 | Protein: 30g | Carbohydrates: 25g | Fat: 18g | Fiber: 4g

3. Turkey and Vegetable Skewers with Mint Yogurt Sauce

Prep Time: 20 minutes

Cooking Time: 15 minutes

Serving Size: 2

Ingredients:

- 1 lb turkey breast, cut into chunks

- 1 zucchini, sliced

- 1 bell pepper, cut into chunks

- 1 red onion, cut into chunks

- 2 tbsp olive oil

- 1 tsp ground cumin

- 1 tsp smoked paprika

- Salt and pepper to taste

Mint Yogurt Sauce:

- 1/2 cup Greek yogurt

- 2 tbsp fresh mint, chopped

- 1 tbsp lemon juice

- 1 garlic clove, minced

- Salt and pepper to taste

Instructions:

1. Preheat the grill or grill pan.

2. In a bowl, toss turkey chunks, sliced zucchini, bell pepper, and red onion with olive oil, ground cumin, smoked paprika, salt, and pepper.

3. Thread the marinated turkey and vegetables onto skewers.

4. Grill for 10-12 minutes, turning occasionally, until turkey is cooked through and vegetables are tender.

5. For the mint yogurt sauce, mix together Greek yogurt, chopped mint, lemon juice, minced garlic, salt, and pepper.

6. Serve the turkey skewers with the mint yogurt sauce.

Nutritional Information:

Calories: 400 | Protein: 35g | Carbohydrates: 15g | Fat: 20g | Fiber: 4g

4. Baked Eggplant Parmesan

Prep Time: 30 minutes

Cooking Time: 25 minutes

Serving Size: 2

Ingredients:

- 1 large eggplant, sliced into rounds

- 1 cup whole wheat breadcrumbs

- 1/2 cup grated Parmesan cheese

- 2 eggs, beaten

- 2 cups marinara sauce

- 1 cup part-skim mozzarella cheese, shredded

- Fresh basil for garnish

Instructions:

1. Preheat the oven to 400°F (200°C).

2. Dip eggplant slices in beaten eggs, then coat with a mixture of whole wheat breadcrumbs and grated Parmesan.

3. Place the coated eggplant slices on a baking sheet and bake for 15-20 minutes or until golden brown.

4. In a baking dish, layer marinara sauce, baked eggplant slices, and shredded mozzarella.

5. Repeat the layers and top with mozzarella cheese.

6. Bake for an additional 15 minutes or until the cheese is melted and bubbly.

7. Garnish with fresh basil before serving.

Nutritional Information:

Calories: 380 | Protein: 20g | Carbohydrates: 40g | Fat: 15g | Fiber: 12g

5. Lemon Garlic Shrimp and Asparagus Stir-Fry

Prep Time: 15 minutes

Cooking Time: 10 minutes

Serving Size: 2

Ingredients:

- 1 lb shrimp, peeled and deveined

- 1 bunch asparagus, trimmed and cut into 2-inch pieces

- 2 tbsp olive oil

- 3 garlic cloves, minced

- Zest of 1 lemon

- 2 tbsp fresh lemon juice

- 1/2 tsp red pepper flakes (optional)

- Salt and pepper to taste

Instructions:

1. In a wok or skillet, heat olive oil over medium-high heat.

2. Add shrimp and asparagus, stir-frying until shrimp are pink and opaque.

3. Add minced garlic, lemon zest, lemon juice, red pepper flakes (if using), salt, and pepper. Stir-fry for an additional 2 minutes.

4. Serve the lemon garlic shrimp and asparagus over cooked quinoa or brown rice.

Nutritional Information:

Calories: 320 | Protein: 30g | Carbohydrates: 15g | Fat: 18g | Fiber: 6g

6. Stuffed Bell Peppers with Ground Turkey and Quinoa

Prep Time: 20 minutes

Cooking Time: 30 minutes

Serving Size: 2 peppers

Ingredients:

- 1/2 cup uncooked quinoa

- 1 cup water

- 2 large bell peppers, halved and seeds removed

- 1 lb ground turkey

- 1 onion, chopped

- 1 can (14 oz) diced tomatoes, drained

- 1 tsp cumin

- 1/2 tsp chili powder

- Salt and pepper to taste

- 1/2 cup shredded cheddar cheese

Instructions:

1. Cook quinoa in water according to package instructions.

2. Preheat the oven to 375°F (190°C).

3. In a skillet, brown ground turkey with chopped onion until cooked through.

4. Add cooked quinoa, diced tomatoes, cumin, chili powder, salt, and pepper to the turkey mixture. Stir well.

5. Stuff each bell pepper half with the turkey and quinoa mixture.

6. Top with shredded cheddar cheese.

7. Bake for 25-30 minutes or until peppers are tender and cheese is melted.

Nutritional Information:

Calories: 380 | Protein: 30g | Carbohydrates: 30g | Fat: 15g | Fiber: 6g

7. Spinach and Feta Stuffed Portobello Mushrooms

Prep Time: 20 minutes

Cooking Time: 20 minutes

Serving Size: 2 mushrooms

Ingredients:

- 4 large Portobello mushrooms, stems removed

- 2 cups fresh spinach, chopped

- 1/2 cup feta cheese, crumbled

- 1/4 cup red onion, finely chopped

- 2 tbsp olive oil

- 2 tsp balsamic vinegar

- Salt and pepper to taste

Instructions:

1. Preheat the oven to 375°F (190°C).

2. Place Portobello mushrooms on a baking sheet.

3. In a skillet, sauté chopped spinach, crumbled feta, and finely chopped red onion in olive oil until spinach wilts.

4. Season with balsamic vinegar, salt, and pepper.

5. Spoon the spinach and feta mixture into each Portobello mushroom.

6. Bake for 20 minutes or until mushrooms are tender.

Nutritional Information:

Calories: 340 | Protein: 15g | Carbohydrates: 20g | Fat: 18g | Fiber: 6g

8. Teriyaki Turkey and Vegetable Stir-Fry

Prep Time: 15 minutes

Cooking Time: 15 minutes

Serving Size: 2

Ingredients:

- 1 lb ground turkey

- 1 cup broccoli florets

- 1 bell pepper, sliced

- 1 carrot, julienned

- 1 cup snap peas

- 1/4 cup low-sodium teriyaki sauce

- 2 tbsp soy sauce

- 1 tbsp sesame oil

- 1 tbsp rice vinegar

- 1 tbsp fresh ginger, grated

- 2 garlic cloves, minced

- 2 green onions, sliced

Instructions:

1. In a wok or skillet, brown ground turkey until cooked through.

2. Add broccoli, bell pepper, julienned carrot, and snap peas. Stir-fry until vegetables are crisp-tender.

3. In a small bowl, whisk together teriyaki sauce, soy sauce, sesame oil, rice vinegar, grated ginger, and minced garlic.

4. Pour the sauce over the turkey and vegetable mixture, toss until well coated.

5. Garnish with sliced green onions before serving.

Nutritional Information:

Calories: 350 | Protein: 25g | Carbohydrates: 25g | Fat: 18g | Fiber: 6g

9. Mediterranean Baked Cod with Tomato and Olive Relish

Prep Time: 15 minutes

Cooking Time: 20 minutes

Serving Size: 2

Ingredients:

- 2 cod fillets

- 1 cup cherry tomatoes, halved

- 1/4 cup Kalamata olives, pitted and sliced

- 2 tbsp fresh parsley, chopped

- 2 tbsp olive oil

- 1 tbsp capers

- 1 tsp dried oregano

- Salt and pepper to taste

Instructions:

1. Preheat the oven to 400°F (200°C).

2. Place cod fillets on a baking sheet.

3. In a bowl, mix cherry tomatoes, sliced Kalamata olives, chopped fresh parsley, olive oil, capers, dried oregano, salt, and pepper.

4. Spoon the tomato and olive relish over the cod fillets.

5. Bake for 20 minutes or until the fish is opaque and flakes easily.

Nutritional Information:

Calories: 320 | Protein: 30g | Carbohydrates: 10g | Fat: 18g | Fiber: 3g

10. Chickpea and Vegetable Curry with Brown Rice

Prep Time: 20 minutes
Cooking Time: 30 minutes
Serving Size: 2

Ingredients:

- 1 can (14 oz) chickpeas, drained and rinsed

- 1 cup cauliflower florets

- 1 cup sweet potatoes, diced

- 1 cup cherry tomatoes, halved

- 1 onion, chopped

- 2 tbsp curry powder

- 1 tsp ground turmeric

- 1 tsp cumin

- 1 can (14 oz) coconut milk

- 1 cup cooked brown rice

- Fresh cilantro for garnish

Instructions:

1. In a pot, sauté chopped onion until softened.

2. Add chickpeas, cauliflower, sweet potatoes, cherry tomatoes, curry powder, ground turmeric, and cumin. Stir well.

3. Pour in coconut milk and simmer for 25-30 minutes or until vegetables are tender.

4. Serve the chickpea and vegetable curry over cooked brown rice.

5. Garnish with fresh cilantro before serving.

Nutritional Information:

Calories: 380 | Protein: 15g | Carbohydrates: 50g | Fat: 15g | Fiber: 12g

11. Lemon Herb Grilled Chicken Breast with Quinoa Salad

Prep Time: 15 minutes

Cooking Time: 15 minutes

Serving Size: 2

Ingredients:

- 2 boneless, skinless chicken breasts

- 1 cup cooked quinoa

- 1 cucumber, diced

- 1 cup cherry tomatoes, halved

- 1/4 cup red onion, finely chopped

- 2 tbsp fresh parsley, chopped

- 2 tbsp olive oil

- Zest and juice of 1 lemon

- Salt and pepper to taste

Instructions:

1. Preheat the grill or grill pan.

2. Season chicken breasts with salt, pepper, and olive oil.

3. Grill chicken for 6-8 minutes per side or until cooked through.

4. In a bowl, combine cooked quinoa, diced cucumber, cherry tomatoes, chopped red onion, chopped fresh parsley, olive oil, lemon zest, lemon juice, salt, and pepper.

5. Serve the grilled chicken over the quinoa salad.

Nutritional Information:

Calories: 340 | Protein: 30g | Carbohydrates: 30g | Fat: 15g | Fiber: 6g

12. Baked Turkey Meatballs with Zucchini Noodles

Prep Time: 20 minutes

Cooking Time: 25 minutes

Serving Size: 2

Ingredients:

- 1 lb ground turkey

- 1/2 cup whole wheat breadcrumbs

- 1/4 cup grated Parmesan cheese

- 1 egg

- 2 garlic cloves, minced

- 1 tsp dried oregano

- 1/2 tsp red pepper flakes (optional)

- Salt and pepper to taste

Zucchini Noodles:

- 2 zucchinis, spiralized

- 1 tbsp olive oil

- 1 garlic clove, minced

- 1/4 cup fresh basil, chopped

Instructions:

1. Preheat the oven to 400°F (200°C).

2. In a bowl, mix ground turkey, whole wheat breadcrumbs, grated Parmesan, egg, minced garlic, dried oregano, red pepper flakes (if using), salt, and pepper.

3. Form the mixture into meatballs and place them on a baking sheet.

4. Bake for 20-25 minutes or until the meatballs are cooked through.

5. In a skillet, heat olive oil and sauté spiralized zucchini with minced garlic for 2-3 minutes.

6. Toss zucchini noodles with fresh basil and serve with the turkey meatballs.

Nutritional Information:

Calories: 360 | Protein: 30g | Carbohydrates: 20g | Fat: 18g | Fiber: 4g

13. Shrimp and Broccoli Stir-Fry with Brown Rice

Prep Time: 15 minutes

Cooking Time: 15 minutes

Serving Size: 2

Ingredients:

- 1 lb shrimp, peeled and deveined

- 2 cups broccoli florets

- 1 bell pepper, sliced

- 1 cup snap peas

- 2 tbsp soy sauce

- 1 tbsp oyster sauce

- 1 tbsp sesame oil

- 1 tbsp rice vinegar

- 2 garlic cloves, minced

- 1 tsp ginger, grated

- 2 cups cooked brown rice

Instructions:

1. In a wok or skillet, stir-fry shrimp, broccoli, bell pepper, and snap peas until shrimp are pink and opaque.

2. In a small bowl, whisk together soy sauce, oyster sauce, sesame oil, rice vinegar, minced garlic, and grated ginger.

3. Add the sauce to the stir-fry and toss until well coated.

4. Serve the shrimp and broccoli stir-fry over cooked brown rice.

Nutritional Information:

Calories: 380 | Protein: 30g | Carbohydrates: 45g | Fat: 15g | Fiber: 8g

14. Grilled Vegetable and Chicken Skewers with Pesto Sauce

Prep Time: 20 minutes

Cooking Time: 15 minutes

Serving Size: 2

Ingredients:

- 1 lb chicken breast, cut into chunks

- 1 zucchini, sliced

- 1 yellow bell pepper, cut into chunks

- 1 red onion, cut into chunks

- 1 cup cherry tomatoes

- 2 tbsp olive oil

- Salt and pepper to taste

Pesto Sauce:

- 2 cups fresh basil leaves

- 1/2 cup grated Parmesan cheese

- 1/2 cup pine nuts

- 2 garlic cloves

- 1/2 cup olive oil

- Salt and pepper to taste

Instructions:

1. Preheat the grill or grill pan.

2. In a bowl, toss chicken chunks, sliced zucchini, bell pepper, red onion, and cherry tomatoes with olive oil, salt, and pepper.

3. Thread the marinated chicken and vegetables onto skewers.

4. Grill for 10-12 minutes, turning occasionally, until chicken is cooked through and vegetables are tender.

5. For the pesto sauce, blend basil leaves, Parmesan cheese, pine nuts, garlic cloves, and olive oil until smooth. Season with salt and pepper.

6. Serve the grilled skewers with a side of pesto sauce.

Nutritional Information:

Calories: 420 | Protein: 35g | Carbohydrates: 15g | Fat: 25g | Fiber: 4g

15. Spaghetti Squash with Turkey Bolognese

Prep Time: 20 minutes

Cooking Time: 45 minutes

Serving Size: 2

Ingredients:

- 1 spaghetti squash, halved and seeds removed

- 1 lb ground turkey

- 1 onion, chopped

- 2 carrots, diced

- 2 celery stalks, diced

- 2 garlic cloves, minced

- 1 can (14 oz) crushed tomatoes

- 1 tsp dried oregano

- 1 tsp dried basil

- Salt and pepper to taste

Instructions:

1. Preheat the oven to 400°F (200°C).

2. Place spaghetti squash halves on a baking sheet, cut side down.

3. Bake for 30-40 minutes or until the squash is tender and easily shredded with a fork.

4. In a skillet, brown ground turkey with chopped onion, diced carrots, diced celery, and minced garlic.

5. Add crushed tomatoes, dried oregano, dried basil, salt, and pepper to the turkey mixture. Simmer for 15-20 minutes.

6. Shred the cooked spaghetti squash with a fork and serve topped with turkey Bolognese.

Nutritional Information:

Calories: 380 | Protein: 30g | Carbohydrates: 35g | Fat: 18g | Fiber: 10g

16. Baked Halibut with Lemon Caper Sauce and Steamed Asparagus

Prep Time: 15 minutes

Cooking Time: 20 minutes

Serving Size: 2

Ingredients:

- 2 halibut fillets

- 1 bunch asparagus, trimmed

- 2 tbsp olive oil

- 2 tbsp capers

- 1/4 cup fresh lemon juice

- 1 tsp Dijon mustard

- 2 tbsp fresh parsley, chopped

- Salt and pepper to taste

Instructions:

1. Preheat the oven to 400°F (200°C).

2. Place halibut fillets on a baking sheet.

3. Drizzle olive oil over the halibut and season with salt and pepper.

4. Bake for 15-20 minutes or until the fish is opaque and flakes easily.

5. In a small saucepan, combine capers, fresh lemon juice, Dijon mustard, and chopped fresh parsley. Heat over low heat until warmed.

6. Steam asparagus until tender-crisp.

7. Serve the baked halibut over steamed asparagus, drizzled with lemon caper sauce.

Nutritional Information:

Calories: 320 | Protein: 30g | Carbohydrates: 10g | Fat: 18g | Fiber: 4g

17. Lentil and Vegetable Stuffed Peppers

Prep Time: 25 minutes

Cooking Time: 30 minutes

Serving Size: 2 peppers

Ingredients:

- 1 cup dried green lentils

- 2 cups water

- 4 large bell peppers, halved and seeds removed

- 1 onion, chopped

- 2 carrots, diced

- 2 celery stalks, diced

- 2 garlic cloves, minced

- 1 can (14 oz) diced tomatoes, drained

- 1 tsp ground cumin

- 1 tsp smoked paprika

- Salt and pepper to taste

- 1/2 cup feta cheese, crumbled

Instructions:

1. Cook lentils in water according to package instructions.

2. Preheat the oven to 375°F (190°C).

3. In a skillet, sauté chopped onion, diced carrots, diced celery, and minced garlic until softened.

4. Add cooked lentils, drained diced tomatoes, ground cumin, smoked paprika, salt, and pepper. Stir well.

5. Stuff each bell pepper half with the lentil and vegetable mixture.

6. Top with crumbled feta cheese.

7. Bake for 25-30 minutes or until peppers are tender.

Nutritional Information:

Calories: 380 | Protein: 20g | Carbohydrates: 55g | Fat: 10g | Fiber: 15g

18. Chicken and Vegetable Brown Rice Bowl

Prep Time: 15 minutes

Cooking Time: 20 minutes

Serving Size: 2

Ingredients:

- 2 boneless, skinless chicken breasts

- 1 cup broccoli florets

- 1 bell pepper, sliced

- 1 carrot, julienned

- 2 cups cooked brown rice

- 2 tbsp low-sodium soy sauce

- 1 tbsp hoisin sauce

- 1 tbsp sesame oil

- 1 tsp fresh ginger, grated

- 2 garlic cloves, minced

- Green onions for garnish

Instructions:

1. Season chicken breasts with salt and pepper.

2. Grill or cook chicken in a skillet until cooked through.

3. In the same skillet, stir-fry broccoli, bell pepper, and julienned carrot until crisp-tender.

4. Slice the cooked chicken and add it to the vegetable mixture.

5. In a small bowl, whisk together soy sauce, hoisin sauce, sesame oil, grated ginger, and minced garlic.

6. Pour the sauce over the chicken and vegetables, toss until well coated.

7. Serve the chicken and vegetable stir-fry over cooked brown rice, garnished with green onions.

Nutritional Information:

Calories: 400 | Protein: 35g | Carbohydrates: 50g | Fat: 10g | Fiber: 8g

19. Moroccan Spiced Chickpea and Vegetable Tagine

Prep Time: 25 minutes

Cooking Time: 30 minutes

Serving Size: 2

Ingredients:

- 1 can (14 oz) chickpeas, drained and rinsed

- 1 eggplant, diced

- 1 zucchini, diced

- 1 bell pepper, diced

- 1 onion, chopped

- 2 garlic cloves, minced

- 1 can (14 oz) diced tomatoes

- 1/2 cup vegetable broth

- 2 tsp ground cumin

- 1 tsp ground coriander

- 1 tsp smoked paprika

- 1/2 tsp ground cinnamon

- Salt and pepper to taste

- Fresh cilantro for garnish

Instructions:

1. In a pot, sauté chopped onion and minced garlic until softened.

2. Add diced eggplant, diced zucchini, diced bell pepper, chickpeas, diced tomatoes, vegetable broth, ground cumin, ground coriander, smoked paprika, ground cinnamon, salt, and pepper. Stir well.

3. Simmer for 25-30 minutes or until vegetables are tender.

4. Garnish with fresh cilantro before serving.

Nutritional Information:

Calories: 360 | Protein: 15g | Carbohydrates: 65g | Fat: 8g | Fiber: 18g

20. Teriyaki Glazed Salmon with Quinoa and Steamed Green Beans

Prep Time: 15 minutes

Cooking Time: 15 minutes

Serving Size: 2

Ingredients:

- 2 salmon fillets

- 1 cup quinoa, cooked

- 1 lb green beans, trimmed

- 1/4 cup low-sodium teriyaki sauce

- 1 tbsp honey

- 1 tbsp rice vinegar

- 1 tsp sesame oil

- 1 tsp fresh ginger, grated

- Sesame seeds for garnish

Instructions:

1. Preheat the oven to 400°F (200°C).

2. Place salmon fillets on a baking sheet.

3. In a small bowl, whisk together teriyaki sauce, honey, rice vinegar, sesame oil, and grated ginger.

4. Brush the teriyaki glaze over the salmon fillets.

5. Bake for 12-15 minutes or until the salmon is cooked through.

6. Steam green beans until tender-crisp.

7. Serve the teriyaki glazed salmon over cooked quinoa, garnished with sesame seeds.

Nutritional Information:

Calories: 420 | Protein: 30g | Carbohydrates: 40g | Fat: 18g | Fiber: 8g

SNACKS RECIPES

1. Greek Yogurt and Berry Parfait

Prep Time: 10 minutes

Serving Size: 1

Ingredients:

- 1 cup Greek yogurt
- 1/2 cup mixed berries (blueberries, strawberries, raspberries)
- 2 tbsp honey
- 1/4 cup granola

Instructions:

1. In a glass or bowl, layer Greek yogurt, mixed berries, and granola.
2. Drizzle honey over the top.
3. Repeat the layers.
4. Serve immediately.

Nutritional Information:

Calories: 250 | Protein: 18g | Carbohydrates: 40g | Fat: 5g | Fiber: 4g

2. Avocado and Hummus Rice Cakes

Prep Time: 5 minutes

Serving Size: 2 rice cakes

Ingredients:

- 2 rice cakes

- 1 avocado, sliced

- 1/2 cup hummus

- Cherry tomatoes, halved, for garnish

- Fresh parsley, chopped, for garnish

Instructions:

1. Spread a layer of hummus on each rice cake.

2. Top with sliced avocado.

3. Garnish with cherry tomatoes and chopped fresh parsley.

4. Serve immediately.

Nutritional Information:

Calories: 280 | Protein: 8g | Carbohydrates: 25g | Fat: 18g | Fiber: 8g

3. Cucumber and Smoked Salmon Roll-Ups

Prep Time: 15 minutes

Serving Size: 4 rolls

Ingredients:

- 1 large cucumber

- 4 oz smoked salmon

- 1/4 cup cream cheese

- Fresh dill, for garnish

Instructions:

1. Using a vegetable peeler, slice the cucumber into thin strips.

2. Spread a layer of cream cheese on each cucumber strip.

3. Place a piece of smoked salmon on top of the cream cheese.

4. Roll up the cucumber strips with the smoked salmon.

5. Garnish with fresh dill.

6. Serve chilled.

Nutritional Information:

Calories: 180 | Protein: 15g | Carbohydrates: 5g | Fat: 10g | Fiber: 1g

4. Almond Butter and Banana Rice Cakes

Prep Time: 5 minutes

Serving Size: 2 rice cakes

Ingredients:

- 2 rice cakes

- 1/4 cup almond butter

- 1 banana, sliced

- Chia seeds, for garnish

Instructions:

1. Spread a layer of almond butter on each rice cake.

2. Top with sliced banana.

3. Sprinkle chia seeds over the top.

4. Serve immediately.

Nutritional Information:

Calories: 320 | Protein: 7g | Carbohydrates: 35g | Fat: 18g | Fiber: 6g

5. Quinoa and Veggie Stuffed Bell Peppers

Prep Time: 15 minutes

Cooking Time: 0 minutes (no cooking required)

Serving Size: 2 peppers

Ingredients:

- 2 bell peppers, halved and seeds removed

- 1 cup cooked quinoa

- 1/2 cup cherry tomatoes, diced

- 1/4 cup cucumber, diced

- 1/4 cup feta cheese, crumbled

- Fresh mint, chopped, for garnish

Instructions:

1. In a bowl, mix together cooked quinoa, diced cherry tomatoes, diced cucumber, and crumbled feta.

2. Spoon the quinoa mixture into each bell pepper half.

3. Garnish with fresh mint.

4. Serve chilled.

Nutritional Information:

Calories: 280 | Protein: 10g | Carbohydrates: 40g | Fat: 10g | Fiber: 6g

6. Apple Slices with Almond Butter and Walnuts

Prep Time: 10 minutes

Serving Size: 1

Ingredients:

- 1 apple, sliced

- 2 tbsp almond butter

- 1/4 cup walnuts, chopped

Instructions:

1. Spread almond butter on each apple slice.

2. Sprinkle chopped walnuts over the almond butter.

3. Serve immediately.

Nutritional Information:

Calories: 230 | Protein: 5g | Carbohydrates: 20g | Fat: 15g | Fiber: 5g

7. Edamame and Sea Salt Snack Bowl

Prep Time: 5 minutes

Cooking Time: 5 minutes (if using frozen edamame)

Serving Size: 1

Ingredients:

- 1 cup edamame (fresh or frozen)

- Sea salt, to taste

Instructions:

1. If using frozen edamame, cook according to package instructions.

2. Sprinkle sea salt over the edamame.

3. Toss to coat.

4. Serve chilled.

Nutritional Information:

Calories: 180 | Protein: 17g | Carbohydrates: 14g | Fat: 8g | Fiber: 8g

8. Roasted Chickpeas with Turmeric and Cumin

Prep Time: 10 minutes

Cooking Time: 25 minutes

Serving Size: 1/2 cup

Ingredients:

- 1 can (14 oz) chickpeas, drained and rinsed

- 1 tbsp olive oil

- 1 tsp ground turmeric

- 1 tsp ground cumin

- Salt and pepper to taste

Instructions:

1. Preheat the oven to 400°F (200°C).

2. In a bowl, toss chickpeas with olive oil, ground turmeric, ground cumin, salt, and pepper.

3. Spread the chickpeas on a baking sheet.

4. Roast for 25 minutes or until crispy.

5. Allow to cool before serving.

Nutritional Information:

Calories: 220 | Protein: 10g | Carbohydrates: 30g | Fat: 8g | Fiber: 7g

9. Cottage Cheese and Pineapple Bowl

Prep Time: 5 minutes

Serving Size: 1

Ingredients:

- 1 cup low-fat cottage cheese

- 1/2 cup fresh pineapple chunks

- 1 tbsp flaxseeds

Instructions:

1. In a bowl, combine cottage cheese and fresh pineapple chunks.

2. Sprinkle flaxseeds over the top.

3. Serve chilled.

Nutritional Information:

Calories: 220 | Protein: 25g | Carbohydrates: 20g | Fat: 6g | Fiber: 3g

10. Turkey and Cheese Lettuce Wraps

Prep Time: 10 minutes

Serving Size: 2 wraps

Ingredients:

- 4 large lettuce leaves (iceberg or romaine)

- 6 oz turkey breast slices

- 2 slices Swiss cheese

- Dijon mustard, for drizzling

- 1/4 cup cucumber, julienned

Instructions:

1. Lay out the lettuce leaves.

2. Place turkey breast slices on each leaf.

3. Add a slice of Swiss cheese to each.

4. Drizzle with Dijon mustard and top with julienned cucumber.

5. Roll up the lettuce leaves to form wraps.

6. Serve chilled.

Nutritional Information:

Calories: 280 | Protein: 30g | Carbohydrates: 5g | Fat: 15g | Fiber: 2g

DESSERT RECIPES

1. Berry and Greek Yogurt Parfait

Prep Time: 10 minutes

Cooking Time: 0 minutes

Serving Size: 1 parfait

Ingredients:

- 1 cup mixed berries (blueberries, strawberries, raspberries)

- 1 cup Greek yogurt

- 2 tbsp honey

- 1/4 cup granola

Instructions:

1. In a glass, layer mixed berries, Greek yogurt, and granola.

2. Drizzle honey over the top.

3. Repeat the layers.

4. Serve immediately.

Nutritional Information:

Calories: 250 | Protein: 18g | Carbohydrates: 40g | Fat: 5g | Fiber: 4g

2. Dark Chocolate-Dipped Strawberries

Prep Time: 15 minutes

Cooking Time: 5 minutes

Serving Size: 2 strawberries

Ingredients:

- 1 cup dark chocolate chips

- 12 large strawberries, washed and dried

Instructions:

1. Melt dark chocolate chips in a microwave-safe bowl in 30-second intervals, stirring between each interval until smooth.

2. Dip each strawberry into the melted chocolate, covering about two-thirds of the strawberry.

3. Place the dipped strawberries on a parchment-lined tray.

4. Refrigerate until the chocolate hardens.

5. Serve chilled.

Nutritional Information:

Calories: 120 | Protein: 1g | Carbohydrates: 15g | Fat: 7g | Fiber: 3g

3. Baked Apples with Cinnamon and Walnuts

Prep Time: 15 minutes

Cooking Time: 30 minutes

Serving Size: 1 apple

Ingredients:

- 2 apples, cored and halved

- 1 tbsp lemon juice

- 1 tsp ground cinnamon

- 1/4 cup chopped walnuts

- 1 tbsp honey

Instructions:

1. Preheat the oven to 375°F (190°C).

2. Place apple halves in a baking dish and drizzle with lemon juice.

3. Sprinkle ground cinnamon over the apples and top with chopped walnuts.

4. Drizzle honey over the top.

5. Bake for 30 minutes or until apples are tender.

6. Serve warm.

Nutritional Information:

Calories: 200 | Protein: 2g | Carbohydrates: 30g | Fat: 10g | Fiber: 6g

4. Chia Seed Pudding with Mango

Prep Time: 5 minutes (plus overnight refrigeration)

Cooking Time: 0 minutes

Serving Size: 1 pudding

Ingredients:

- 2 tbsp chia seeds

- 1/2 cup almond milk

- 1/2 tsp vanilla extract

- 1 tbsp maple syrup

- 1/2 cup diced mango

Instructions:

1. In a jar, combine chia seeds, almond milk, vanilla extract, and maple syrup.

2. Stir well, cover, and refrigerate overnight.

3. In the morning, stir the chia pudding and top with diced mango.

4. Serve chilled.

Nutritional Information:

Calories: 220 | Protein: 5g | Carbohydrates: 30g | Fat: 10g | Fiber: 10g

5. Frozen Banana and Almond Butter Bites

Prep Time: 10 minutes

Cooking Time: 0 minutes (freezing time)

Serving Size: 4 bites

Ingredients:

- 2 bananas, sliced

- 1/4 cup almond butter

- 1/4 cup chopped almonds

Instructions:

1. Spread almond butter on one side of each banana slice.

2. Sandwich two banana slices together, creating bites.

3. Roll the edges of the bites in chopped almonds.

4. Place the bites on a tray and freeze until solid.

5. Serve frozen.

Nutritional Information:

Calories: 180 | Protein: 4g | Carbohydrates: 20g | Fat: 10g | Fiber: 4g

6. Lemon Sorbet with Mint

Prep Time: 10 minutes

Cooking Time: 0 minutes (freezing time)

Serving Size: 1 scoop

Ingredients:

- 2 cups frozen lemon segments

- 1/4 cup fresh mint leaves

- 2 tbsp honey

Instructions:

1. In a blender, combine frozen lemon segments, fresh mint leaves, and honey.

2. Blend until smooth and creamy.

3. Transfer the sorbet mixture to a container and freeze until firm.

4. Scoop and serve.

Nutritional Information:

Calories: 150 | Protein: 1g | Carbohydrates: 40g | Fat: 0g | Fiber: 5g

7. Peach and Oat Crisp

Prep Time: 15 minutes

Cooking Time: 30 minutes

Serving Size: 1 serving

Ingredients:

- 1 cup sliced peaches (fresh or frozen)

- 1/4 cup rolled oats

- 2 tbsp almond flour

- 1 tbsp honey

- 1/2 tsp ground cinnamon

- 1 tbsp chopped almonds

Instructions:

1. Preheat the oven to 350°F (180°C).

2. In a bowl, mix sliced peaches with rolled oats, almond flour, honey, and ground cinnamon.

3. Transfer the mixture to a baking dish.

4. Sprinkle chopped almonds over the top.

5. Bake for 30 minutes or until the top is golden and the peaches are bubbling.

6. Serve warm.

Nutritional Information:

Calories: 220 | Protein: 4g | Carbohydrates: 40g | Fat: 7g | Fiber: 6g

8. Coconut Milk Rice Pudding

Prep Time: 10 minutes

Cooking Time: 30 minutes

Serving Size: 1/2 cup

Ingredients:

- 1/2 cup Arborio rice

- 1 can (14 oz) coconut milk

- 1/4 cup maple syrup

- 1/2 tsp vanilla extract

- 1/4 cup shredded coconut

Instructions:

1. In a saucepan, combine Arborio rice, coconut milk, maple syrup, and vanilla extract.

2. Bring to a simmer and cook for 25-30 minutes, stirring occasionally, until the rice is tender.

3. Stir in shredded coconut.

4. Remove from heat and let it cool.

5. Serve chilled.

Nutritional Information:

Calories: 300 | Protein: 3g | Carbohydrates: 35g | Fat: 17g | Fiber: 1g

9. Raspberry and Almond Crumble Bars

Prep Time: 20 minutes

Cooking Time: 30 minutes

Serving Size: 1 bar

Ingredients:

- 1 cup fresh or frozen raspberries

- 1 cup almond flour

- 1/4 cup coconut oil, melted

- 2 tbsp maple syrup

- 1/2 cup sliced almonds

Instructions:

1. Preheat the oven to 350°F (180°C).

2. In a bowl, mix almond flour, melted coconut oil, and maple syrup to form a crumbly mixture.

3. Press half of the mixture into a baking dish to create the base.

4. Spread raspberries over the base.

5. Sprinkle the remaining crumbly mixture and sliced almonds over the top.

6. Bake for 30 minutes or until the top is golden.

7. Allow to cool before slicing.

Nutritional Information:

Calories: 260 | Protein: 6g | Carbohydrates: 20g | Fat: 18g | Fiber: 5g

10. Watermelon and Mint Salad

Prep Time: 15 minutes

Cooking Time: 0 minutes

Serving Size: 1 cup

Ingredients:

- 2 cups cubed watermelon

- 1 tbsp fresh mint leaves, chopped

- 1 tbsp lime juice

- 1 tsp honey

Instructions:

1. In a bowl, combine cubed watermelon and chopped fresh mint.

2. Drizzle lime juice and honey over the top.

3. Toss gently to coat.

4. Serve chilled.

Nutritional Information:

Calories: 80 | Protein: 1g | Carbohydrates: 20g | Fat: 0g | Fiber: 1g

BEVERAGES

Hydrating Choices for Gallbladder Support

Proper hydration is fundamental for maintaining overall health, and it plays a crucial role in supporting gallbladder function. When it comes to choosing beverages for gallbladder support, opting for hydrating choices is essential. Water is the primary hero in this category. It not only helps in keeping the body well-hydrated but also assists in the smooth functioning of the gallbladder.

Water is a natural detoxifier, aiding in the elimination of waste and toxins from the body. Proper hydration also prevents the bile from becoming too concentrated, reducing the risk of gallstone formation. Aim to drink at least eight glasses of water per day, and adjust the intake based on factors like climate, physical activity, and individual needs.

In addition to plain water, incorporating hydrating foods into your diet is another effective way to support gallbladder health. Foods with high water content, such as watermelon, cucumber, and celery, contribute to overall hydration levels. Including these foods in your diet complements the hydrating benefits of water, ensuring that your body stays well-nourished and your gallbladder functions optimally.

For a refreshing twist, infuse your water with slices of fruits like lemon or cucumber. This not only enhances the flavor but also adds a subtle nutritional boost. Herbal infusions, discussed in more detail below, can also be a flavorful and hydrating choice. By making mindful choices about your daily beverages, you contribute to the overall well-being of your gallbladder.

Herbal Teas and Infusions

Herbal teas and infusions offer a comforting and flavorful alternative to traditional caffeinated beverages. When it comes to gallbladder health, certain herbs can provide specific benefits. Peppermint tea, for example, has been associated with relieving digestive discomfort and may help alleviate symptoms of indigestion and bloating.

Ginger tea is another herbal option that has been traditionally used to ease digestive issues. It possesses anti-inflammatory properties that may contribute to a soothing effect on the digestive system. Chamomile tea, known for its calming properties, can be beneficial for relaxation and may indirectly support gallbladder health by promoting overall digestive well-being.

Dandelion root tea is often recommended for its potential to stimulate bile production, aiding in digestion. Bile plays a crucial role in the breakdown of fats, and maintaining a healthy bile flow is essential for gallbladder function. While these herbal teas offer potential benefits, it's advisable to consult with a healthcare professional before incorporating them into your routine, especially if you have pre-existing health conditions or are taking medications.

In addition to herbal teas, infusions with ingredients like fresh mint, rosemary, or basil can be a delightful way to enhance your hydration routine. Experimenting with various flavors not only makes staying hydrated more enjoyable but also provides an opportunity to benefit from the unique properties of different herbs.

It's important to note that while herbal teas and infusions can be a valuable addition to a gallbladder-friendly diet, moderation is key. Excessive consumption of certain herbs may have unintended consequences, and it's advisable to rotate between different varieties to ensure a balanced approach.

Limiting Caffeine and Alcohol

While a moderate amount of caffeine and alcohol consumption is generally considered acceptable for many individuals, those with gallbladder issues may benefit from limiting their intake. Caffeine, commonly found in coffee, tea, and some soft drinks, can stimulate the gallbladder to contract. While this can be a normal response, for individuals prone to gallbladder issues, excessive stimulation may lead to discomfort or exacerbate existing problems.

Opting for decaffeinated versions of coffee and tea is a sensible choice for those looking to reduce their caffeine intake. Herbal teas, as mentioned earlier, offer a caffeine-free alternative with potential additional benefits for gallbladder health. It's essential to pay attention to how your body responds to caffeine and make adjustments based on your individual tolerance and preferences.

Alcohol, on the other hand, can impact the liver, which plays a role in the production and secretion of bile. Excessive alcohol consumption may contribute to liver inflammation and interfere with bile production. Additionally, alcohol can relax the sphincter of Oddi, the muscular valve that controls the flow of bile into the small intestine. This relaxation may result in the reflux of bile back into the gallbladder, potentially causing irritation.

For individuals with gallbladder issues or those at risk, moderation is key. The recommended limits for alcohol consumption vary, but generally, moderate drinking is defined as up to one drink per day for women and up to two drinks per day for men. It's crucial to be mindful of individual health conditions, medications, and any specific recommendations from healthcare providers.

Beverage Recipes

1. Minty Cucumber Infused Water

Prep Time: 5 minutes

Cooking Time: 0 minutes

Serving Size: 1 pitcher (approx. 8 cups)

Ingredients:

- 1 cucumber, thinly sliced

- 1 bunch fresh mint leaves

- 8 cups water

- Ice cubes (optional)

Instructions:

1. In a pitcher, combine sliced cucumber and fresh mint leaves.

2. Fill the pitcher with water.

3. Refrigerate for at least 2 hours to allow flavors to infuse.

4. Serve over ice if desired.

Nutritional Information:

Calories: 0 | Protein: 0g | Carbohydrates: 0g | Fat: 0g | Fiber: 0g

2. Chamomile Ginger Digestive Tea

Prep Time: 5 minutes

Cooking Time: 10 minutes

Serving Size: 1 cup

Ingredients:

- 1 chamomile tea bag

- 1/2-inch fresh ginger, sliced

- 1 tsp honey (optional)

Instructions:

1. Boil water and pour it over the chamomile tea bag in a cup.

2. Add sliced ginger to the cup.

3. Allow the tea to steep for 5-7 minutes.

4. Remove the tea bag and ginger slices.

5. Add honey if desired.

6. Enjoy warm.

Nutritional Information:

Calories: 0 | Protein: 0g | Carbohydrates: 0g | Fat: 0g | Fiber: 0g

3. Berry Basil Infused Sparkling Water

Prep Time: 10 minutes

Cooking Time: 0 minutes

Serving Size: 1 glass

Ingredients:

- 1/2 cup mixed berries (blueberries, raspberries, strawberries)

- 3-4 fresh basil leaves

- Sparkling water

Instructions:

1. Muddle the mixed berries and basil leaves in the bottom of a glass.

2. Fill the glass with sparkling water.

3. Stir gently to combine.

4. Serve over ice if desired.

Nutritional Information:

Calories: 10 | Protein: 0g | Carbohydrates: 2g | Fat: 0g | Fiber: 1g

4. Dandelion Detox Elixir

Prep Time: 5 minutes

Cooking Time: 5 minutes

Serving Size: 1 cup

Ingredients:

- 1 dandelion root tea bag

- 1/2 lemon, juiced

- 1 tsp maple syrup

- 1 pinch cayenne pepper (optional)

Instructions:

1. Brew dandelion root tea in a cup of hot water.

2. Add freshly squeezed lemon juice to the tea.

3. Stir in maple syrup and cayenne pepper if using.

4. Mix well and enjoy warm.

Nutritional Information:

Calories: 10 | Protein: 0g | Carbohydrates: 3g | Fat: 0g | Fiber: 0g

5. Green Tea Citrus Refresher

Prep Time: 5 minutes

Cooking Time: 3 minutes

Serving Size: 1 cup

Ingredients:

- 1 green tea bag

- 1/2 orange, sliced

- 1 sprig fresh mint

- 1 tsp honey (optional)

Instructions:

1. Steep the green tea bag in hot water for 2-3 minutes.

2. Remove the tea bag and let the tea cool to room temperature.

3. Add sliced orange and fresh mint to the tea.

4. Refrigerate for at least 1 hour.

5. Add honey if desired.

6. Serve over ice.

Nutritional Information:

Calories: 10 | Protein: 0g | Carbohydrates: 3g | Fat: 0g | Fiber: 1g

14-DAY MEAL PLAN

Day 1:

- *Breakfast:* Berry and Greek Yogurt Parfait

- *Lunch:* Greek Salad with Grilled Chicken

- *Dinner:* Grilled Lemon Herb Chicken

- *Snack:* Roasted Chickpeas with Turmeric and Cumin

- *Dessert:* Dark Chocolate-Dipped Strawberries

Day 2:

- *Breakfast:* Quinoa and Veggie Stuffed Bell Peppers

- *Lunch:* Quinoa and Black Bean Bowl

- *Dinner:* Baked Salmon with Dill Sauce

- *Snack:* Edamame and Sea Salt Snack Bowl

- *Dessert:* Baked Apples with Cinnamon and Walnuts

Day 3:

- *Breakfast:* Avocado and Hummus Rice Cakes

- *Lunch:* Salmon and Avocado Wrap

- *Dinner:* Vegetable and Tofu Stir-Fry

- *Snack:* Apple Slices with Almond Butter and Walnuts

- *Dessert:* Chia Seed Pudding with Mango

Day 4:

- *Breakfast:* Almond Butter and Banana Rice Cakes

- *Lunch:* Turkey and Vegetable Stir-Fry

- *Dinner:* Quinoa-Stuffed Bell Peppers

- *Snack:* Quinoa and Veggie Stuffed Bell Peppers

- *Dessert:* Frozen Banana and Almond Butter Bites

Day 5:

- *Breakfast:* Quinoa and Veggie Stuffed Bell Peppers

- *Lunch:* Lentil and Vegetable Soup

- *Dinner:* Chicken and Broccoli Casserole

- *Snack:* Cottage Cheese and Pineapple Bowl

- *Dessert:* Lemon Sorbet with Mint

Day 6:

- *Breakfast:* Apple Slices with Almond Butter and Walnuts

- *Lunch:* Spinach and Feta Stuffed Chicken Breast

- *Dinner:* Cauliflower and Chickpea Curry

- *Snack:* Edamame and Sea Salt Snack Bowl

- *Dessert:* Peach and Oat Crisp

Day 7:

- *Breakfast:* Edamame and Sea Salt Snack Bowl

- *Lunch:* Chickpea and Avocado Salad

- *Dinner:* Zucchini Noodles with Pesto

- *Snack:* Turkey and Cheese Lettuce Wraps

- *Dessert:* Coconut Milk Rice Pudding

Day 8:

- *Breakfast:* Roasted Chickpeas with Turmeric and Cumin

- *Lunch:* Shrimp and Broccoli Quinoa Bowl

- *Dinner:* Turkey and Sweet Potato Skillet

- *Snack:* Avocado and Hummus Rice Cakes

- *Dessert:* Raspberry and Almond Crumble Bars

Day 9:

- *Breakfast:* Cottage Cheese and Pineapple Bowl

- *Lunch:* Caprese Salad with Balsamic Glaze

- *Dinner:* Eggplant and Tomato Bake

- *Snack:* Dark Chocolate-Dipped Strawberries

- *Dessert:* Watermelon and Mint Salad

Day 10:

- *Breakfast:* Turkey and Cheese Lettuce Wraps

- *Lunch:* Sweet Potato and Black Bean Quesadilla

- *Dinner:* Lemon Garlic Shrimp Pasta

- *Snack:* Greek Yogurt and Berry Parfait

- *Dessert:* Berry and Greek Yogurt Parfait

Day 11:

- *Breakfast:* Quinoa and Veggie Stuffed Bell Peppers

- *Lunch:* Greek Salad with Grilled Chicken

- *Dinner:* Grilled Lemon Herb Chicken

- *Snack:* Roasted Chickpeas with Turmeric and Cumin

- *Dessert:* Dark Chocolate-Dipped Strawberries

Day 12:

- *Breakfast:* Avocado and Hummus Rice Cakes

- *Lunch:* Salmon and Avocado Wrap

- *Dinner:* Vegetable and Tofu Stir-Fry

- *Snack:* Apple Slices with Almond Butter and Walnuts

- *Dessert:* Baked Apples with Cinnamon and Walnuts

Day 13:

- *Breakfast:* Almond Butter and Banana Rice Cakes

- *Lunch:* Turkey and Vegetable Stir-Fry

- *Dinner:* Quinoa-Stuffed Bell Peppers

- *Snack:* Edamame and Sea Salt Snack Bowl

- *Dessert:* Frozen Banana and Almond Butter Bites

Day 14:

- *Breakfast:* Quinoa and Veggie Stuffed Bell Peppers

- *Lunch:* Lentil and Vegetable Soup

- *Dinner:* Chicken and Broccoli Casserole

- *Snack:* Cottage Cheese and Pineapple Bowl

- *Dessert:* Lemon Sorbet with Mint

CONCLUSION

In wrapping up our journey through the pages of the "Gallbladder Diet Cookbook and Meal Plan," it's clear that taking charge of our health isn't just about what we eat; it's about understanding and nurturing the intricate dance our bodies perform every day. This cookbook isn't just a collection of recipes; it's a companion on the path to gallbladder wellness.

As we delved into the intricacies of the gallbladder and the significance of a gallbladder-friendly diet, the tapestry of our understanding expanded. It became more than just a list of do's and don'ts; it became a guide to crafting a lifestyle that supports our well-being. The importance of incorporating nutrient-rich foods, being mindful of portion sizes, and embracing a variety of flavors painted a vivid picture of how satisfying and enjoyable a gallbladder-friendly diet can be.

The comprehensive exploration of gallbladder diet basics, from understanding the intricacies of the gallbladder diet to practical tips for meal planning, wove together a narrative that goes beyond a mere collection of recipes. It's about building a sustainable and nourishing relationship with the food we eat. The recipes are not just ingredients and instructions; they are invitations to explore the diverse and delectable world of flavors that align with gallbladder health.

Planning our meals became more than just a routine; it became an art. The insights into creating balanced and nutrient-rich meals, understanding the significance of portion control, and the inclusion of sample meal plans for different dietary preferences provided a roadmap. It's like having a friendly guide helping us navigate the realm of gallbladder-friendly choices, making the journey feel less like a chore and more like an exciting exploration of culinary delights.

Special considerations, a section often overlooked, emerged as a beacon of personalized care. The tailored advice for weight management, the nuanced approach to specific health conditions, and the gentle reminder to consult with healthcare professionals added layers of consideration to our gallbladder journey. It emphasized that our bodies are unique, and our paths to wellness should be, too.

And then, we ventured into the realm of snacks, breakfasts, lunches, dinners, and desserts – each recipe a brushstroke in the canvas of a gallbladder-friendly culinary masterpiece. These weren't just meals; they were expressions of creativity, designed to delight our taste buds while respecting the needs of our gallbladders. From hearty breakfasts to savory dinners, each recipe whispered, "You can nourish yourself and enjoy every bite."

As we turn the last page, it's not just a closing chapter; it's a beginning. A beginning of a journey where our choices, flavors, and well-being intertwine. The Gallbladder Diet Cookbook and Meal Plan isn't just a book; it's a companion that walks with us, offering guidance, inspiration, and the assurance that we can savor the journey to gallbladder wellness. So, let's close the book, not on our newfound knowledge, but on the old habits that no longer serve us. Here's to a future of delicious, nourishing choices and a gallbladder that dances to the tune of good health. Cheers to a life well-eaten and well-lived.